# Clinical Judgement and Decision Making for Nursing Students

## Transforming Nursing Practice series

*Transforming Nursing Practice* is the first series of books designed to help students meet the requirements of the NMC Standards and Essential Skills Clusters for degree programmes. Each book addresses a core topic, and together they cover the generic knowledge required for all fields of practice. Accessible and challenging, *Transforming Nursing Practice* helps nursing students prepare for the demands of future healthcare delivery.

## Core knowledge titles:

**Series editor:** Dr Shirley Bach, Head of the School of Nursing and Midwifery at the University of Brighton

| | |
|---|---|
| Communication and Interpersonal Skills in Nursing (2nd edn) | ISBN 978 0 85725 449 8 |
| Contexts of Contemporary Nursing (2nd edn) | ISBN 978 1 84445 374 0 |
| Health Promotion and Public Health for Nursing Students | ISBN 978 0 85725 437 5 |
| Introduction to Medicines Management in Nursing | ISBN 978 1 84445 845 5 |
| Law and Professional Issues in Nursing (2nd edn) | ISBN 978 1 84445 372 6 |
| Leadership, Management and Team Working in Nursing | ISBN 978 0 85725 453 5 |
| Learning Skills for Nursing Students | ISBN 978 1 84445 376 4 |
| Medicines Management in Adult Nursing | ISBN 978 1 84445 842 4 |
| Medicines Management in Children's Nursing | ISBN 978 1 84445 470 9 |
| Medicines Management in Mental Health Nursing | ISBN 978 0 85725 049 0 |
| Nursing Adults with Long Term Conditions | ISBN 978 0 85725 441 2 |
| Nursing and Collaborative Practice (2nd edn) | ISBN 978 1 84445 373 3 |
| Nursing and Mental Health Care | ISBN 978 1 84445 467 9 |
| Passing Calculations Tests for Nursing Students | ISBN 978 1 84445 471 6 |
| Patient and Carer Participation in Nursing | ISBN 978 0 85725 307 1 |
| Successful Practice Learning for Nursing Students (2nd edn) | ISBN 978 0 85725 315 6 |
| What is Nursing? Exploring Theory and Practice (2nd edn) | ISBN 978 0 85725 445 0 |

## Personal and professional learning skills titles:

**Series editors:** Dr Mooi Standing, Principal Lecturer/Professional and International Lead in the Department of Nursing and Applied Clinical Studies, Canterbury Christ Church University and Dr Shirley Bach, Head of the School of Nursing and Midwifery at the University of Brighton

| | |
|---|---|
| Clinical Judgement and Decision Making for Nursing Students | ISBN 978 1 84445 468 6 |
| Critical Thinking and Writing for Nursing Students | ISBN 978 1 84445 366 5 |
| Evidence-based Practice in Nursing | ISBN 978 1 84445 369 6 |
| Information Skills for Nursing Students | ISBN 978 1 84445 381 8 |
| Reflective Practice in Nursing | ISBN 978 1 84445 371 9 |
| Succeeding in Research Project Plans and Literature Reviews for Nursing Students | ISBN 978 0 85725 264 7 |
| Successful Professional Portfolios for Nursing Students | ISBN 978 0 85725 457 3 |
| Understanding Research for Nursing Students | ISBN 978 1 84445 368 9 |

To order, contact our distributor: BEBC Distribution, Albion Close, Parkstone, Poole, BH12 3LL. Telephone: 0845 230 9000, email: learningmatters@bebc.co.uk. You can also find more information on each of these titles and our other learning resources at **www.learning matters.co.uk**. Many of these titles are also available in various e-book formats; please visit our website for more information.

# Clinical Judgement and Decision Making for Nursing Students

Mooi Standing

LearningMatters

First published in 2011 by Learning Matters Ltd

*British Library Cataloguing in Publication Data*
A CIP record for this book is available from the British Library

ISBN: 978 1 84445 468 6

This book is also available in the following ebook formats:

Adobe ebook:    ISBN: 978 1 84445 755 7
ePUB ebook:     ISBN: 978 1 84445 754 0
Kindle:             ISBN: 978 0 85725 018 6

Cover and text design by Toucan Design
Project management by Diana Chambers
Typeset by Kelly Winter
Printed and bound in Great Britain by Short Run Press Ltd, Exeter, Devon

Learning Matters Ltd
20 Cathedral Yard
Exeter EX1 1HB
Tel: 01392 215560
E-mail: info@learningmatters.co.uk
**www.learningmatters.co.uk**

# Contents

# About the author

Dr Mooi Standing is a Principal Lecturer/Professional and International Lead in the Department of Nursing and Applied Clinical Studies, Canterbury Christ Church University.

Mooi practised mental health and general nursing in various hospital and community settings before becoming a lecturer, and has been involved in nurse education for over 20 years. Mooi is actively involved in the development of collaborative nursing programmes at undergraduate and post-qualifying levels internationally. She is the designated Programme Director and Academic Link Manager for the collaborative BSc Nursing Studies with Malaysia. In addition, Mooi teaches and supervises nursing students from undergraduate to PhD level studies.

Mooi is also an accredited Nursing and Midwifery Council (NMC) reviewer/managing reviewer approving, monitoring, and assuring the quality of nursing programmes throughout the United Kingdom. She also provides external consultancy in curriculum development and quality enhancement both nationally and internationally.

# Foreword

Employing our clinical judgement and making decisions about the delivery of care are everyday realities for nurses and nursing students. In this book, Mooi Standing invites the reader to develop a deeper understanding of the processes which underpin our decision-making and make explicit the values, thoughts, attitudes and knowledge which inform and mould the ways in which we go about making clinical, and indeed other forms of, judgements.

This book stands out from the crowd in that it contains a plethora of real and engaging activities which will have meaning and will therefore resonate with all student and trained nurses. It explores ideas, concepts and realities with which we, as nurses, are all perhaps familiar but often find difficult to explain meaningfully.

As with all books in this series, the format of this offering is engaging and fresh. The mix of activity types, the explicit chapter aims and the use of Nursing and Midwifery Council Standards of Competence and Essential Skills Clusters mean the message of each element of every chapter is both clear and demonstrably applicable to nursing practice. That is not to say that the activities are not challenging; they are. The challenge does not lie purely in their academic content but also in the challenges they pose to our preconceived attitudes and opinions, which might so easy colour the ways in which we make decisions and clinical judgements.

The other endearing quality of this book is that its content is not inspired purely by academic endeavours, but by the students who contributed to Mooi Standing's understanding of the ways in which students see the world of clinical decision-making and how this understanding develops through time as a result of experience and reflection both on, and in, practice.

The messages contained within this book are therefore meaningful to both student nurses and those nurses, who like me, are a little more experienced. I both commend and recommend *Clinical Judgement and Decision Making for Nursing Students* to all nursing students and registered nurses who care about how the decisions and judgements they make contribute to the quality of the care.

Jane Abbott, MSc, BA (Hons) RGN. Hospital Director

# Acknowledgements

One of the important themes of this book is that good nursing care depends upon effective collaboration with others. It also applies to writing and I need to thank the following people.

I am indebted to my former students who took part in the research study which inspired and informed this book. I thank them for their openness and reflective, critical self-examination.

I could not have written the book without the infinite patience, rock solid support, contribution in researching case studies, and critical feedback of my beloved husband, Michael Standing.

I wish to thank Professor Emeritus Ken Hammond, University of Colorado for his body of work in decision-making and his generosity and humility in encouraging me to add to it.

Last, but not least, it has been a pleasure to work with Learning Matters in writing this book.

# Introduction

This introduction looks at who should read the book, what it is about, why it is important and how it is structured, and gives a brief overview of the NMC standards and learning activities.

## Who should read the book?

The main audience for this book is pre-registration nursing students of all levels, from beginner to finalist, in each of the Adult, Mental Health, Child and Learning Disabilities fields of practice. It may also be of interest to qualified nurses, clinical mentors and assessors who support students' work-based learning during their practice placements. Lecturers in nursing might find the book a helpful resource for relevant learning or teaching activities.

## What is it about?

The book draws together a wide range of knowledge, skills, attitudes and values that characterise safe and effective clinical judgement and decision-making in nursing. This includes looking at the numerous decisions nurses have to make and the variety of evidence and observations that inform clinical judgement, as well as the different approaches to decision-making according to patients' varying needs, available resources and time constraints. Working through the book will help students to develop their understanding and competence in applying clinical decision-making skills to give the best possible care.

## Why is it important?

Learning about clinical judgement and decision-making is important as it makes us continually question whether our actions are beneficial to patients, and discover and apply better ways of caring for them. Nursing is a practice-based profession, and everything we do affects the health and well-being of those we care for. Nursing practice needs to be safe and effective in promoting health and recovery from illness, and in relieving suffering. Thus, nursing practice and actions need to be well reasoned, responsive to individual needs and evidence-based as appropriate, and to have practical outcomes that benefit patients. We cannot achieve this without exercising sound clinical judgement and decision-making. We are also accountable for the quality of care we provide, and this requires us to explain, justify and defend clinical judgement and decision-making. Reading this book, looking at case studies and doing the activities will help you to integrate theory and practice in clinical judgement and decision-making.

# How is it structured?

The format reflects findings of a research study exploring nursing students' perceptions and experience of clinical decision-making skills from the beginning of their programme to the end of their first year as registered nurses. Ten features/types of clinical decision-making were identified from the research and they provide the focus for Chapters 2–11.

Chapter 1     *What is clinical judgement and decision-making in nursing?* – clarifies terms and shows how all ten types of clinical decision-making are applied to one person's care.

Chapter 2     *Collaborative clinical decision-making* – explores consultation, negotiation and co-operation skills with patients and other health professionals in delivering care.

Chapter 3     *Using observation to inform decisions* – emphasises the importance of what we see or hear as evidence about patients' physical or mental health to inform decisions.

Chapter 4     *Systematic clinical decision-making* – combines critical thinking and problem-solving skills to comprehensively assess, plan, deliver care, review and revise outcomes.

Chapter 5     *Standardised clinical decision-making* – looks at applying local NHS Trust policies and procedures and national evidence-based clinical guidelines to enhance care quality.

Chapter 6     *Prioritising decisions in delivering care* – shows how undertaking risk assessment and management informs the way in which resources are targeted nationally and locally in healthcare.

Chapter 7     *Experience and intuition in decision-making* – looks at the way we accumulate a subconscious repertoire of knowledge and skills that we draw upon when events prompt us to do so.

Chapter 8     *Reflective judgement and decision-making* – helps you to consciously review personal, theoretical and practical understanding of a clinical situation as a guide to future action.

Chapter 9     *Ethical sensitivity in decision-making* – covers respect for patients' human rights of freedom of choice, informed consent, confidentiality, and the need for sensitivity in resolving ethical dilemmas.

Chapter 10     *Accountability for nursing decisions* – identifies who we are answerable to, how we are called to account, and the importance of quality assuring standards of care.

Chapter 11     *Confidence in clinical decision-making* – helps you develop self-assurance and professional assurance to inspire confidence in patients and team members that you can be trusted.

# NMC Standards for Pre-registration Nursing Education and Essential Skills Clusters

The Nursing and Midwifery Council (NMC) has standards of competence that have to be met by applicants to different parts of the nursing and midwifery register. These standards are what the NMC deems necessary for the delivery of safe, effective nursing practice. As well as specific competencies, the NMC identifies specific skills that nursing students must have at various points of their training programme. These Essential Skills Clusters (ESCs) are essential abilities that students need to attain in order to practise to their full potential.

This book identifies some of the competencies and skills within the realm of clinical judgement and decision-making that student nurses need in order to be entered on to the NMC register. These competencies and ESCs are presented at the start of each chapter so that it is clear which of them the chapter addresses. All of the competencies and ESCs in this book relate to the *generic standards* that all nursing students must achieve. This book includes the latest taken from the *Standards for pre-registration nursing education* (NMC, 2010a).

# Learning features

Within each chapter there are points at which you can break to undertake activities, and these are an important element of your understanding of the content of each chapter. You are encouraged, where appropriate, to reflect on your practice and consider how the things you have learned from working with patients might inform your understanding of clinical judgement and decision-making. Other activities will require you to take time away from the book to find out new information that will add to your understanding of the topic under discussion. Some activities challenge you to apply your learning to a question or scenario to help you reflect on issues and practice in more depth. A few activities require you to make observations during your day-to-day life or in the clinical setting. All these activities are designed to increase your understanding of the topics under discussion and how they reflect on nursing practice.

Where appropriate, there are suggested or potential answers to activities at the end of the chapter. It is recommended that you try where possible to engage with the activities in order to increase your understanding of the realities of clinical judgement and decision-making.

A glossary explaining some of the more technical terms can be found at the back of the book. Terms included in the glossary will be in bold type the first time they appear.

# Chapter 1
# What is clinical judgement and decision-making in nursing?

## Chapter aims

By the end of this chapter, you should be able to:

- explain clinical judgement and decision-making in nursing;
- relate intuition, reflection and critical thinking to clinical judgement;
- apply relevant judgement in emergency and planned decision-making;
- understand key concepts of nursing in our professional development;
- explain decision-making criteria – practicality, logic, relevance and rigour;
- apply ten types of clinical decision-making to a vulnerable patient's case study..

# Introduction

The purpose of this chapter is to explain what **clinical judgement and decision-making** in **nursing** means and to stimulate your interest in reading the remainder of the book. It gives you a taste of what is to come in the way it uses case studies to help bring the subject to life and activities to help you to relate theory to your own experience and clinical practice. Collectively, the case studies used in this book are applicable to the full range of pre-registration nursing pathways (Adult, Child, Mental Health and Learning Disabilities). Case studies are a good way to explore decision-making, as the following case study illustrates.

## Case study: Car crash

*Roger, aged 44, is about to go and pick up his son from university for the Christmas vacation. It is a cold day and the sky is overcast, but it is dry. Roger is aware there have been reports of snow in other parts of the country, expected to move his way by nightfall. He decides to set off early enough to complete the 220-mile return journey before it gets dark. Twenty minutes into the journey it begins to snow heavily, gritting lorries are working to prevent it from settling on the motorway but two lanes are already covered in 5cm of snow. Roger has experience of driving in these conditions, so although he is surprised by it coming so early, he chooses to carry on. He sees a 50mph speed restriction is enforced and checks how fast he is going (45mph). He is following a lorry. He cannot see that further up the road a car has skidded into the crash barrier. The back of the lorry is thick with dirt and snow, and Roger is unable to see that its brake lights are on. He suddenly realises he is going to smash into the lorry.*

*Roger takes his foot off the accelerator and changes to a lower gear, but the wheels do not grip and he does not slow down enough. He frantically 'pumps' the foot brake to try to slow down without skidding but it is too late. He is half a second away from driving into the back of the lorry. In desperation he steers the car away and tries to thread his way through traffic in the inner lane but the steering is not very responsive in such slippery conditions. Roger collides with one car and is hit by another, all the airbags are deployed, and front and rear windscreens are broken by the force of impact. He manages to stop the car on the hard shoulder. The car is a 'write off' (damaged beyond economical repair), and Roger is badly shaken up. The car that was behind him ploughs into the back of the lorry, and the driver is treated for neck injuries. A police investigation rules that no one can be held responsible for what happened.*

There were no fatalities associated with the case study, but road traffic accidents in the UK claim on average 3,000 lives each year (Office for National Statistics, 2006). It is possible that Roger escaped serious injury by avoiding contact with both the lorry in front of him and the car behind him.

Although the police ruled out prosecuting anyone for causing the accident by dangerous driving, it is still important to look at how the accident might have been prevented to inform future road safety. Activity 1.1 asks you some questions to explore this further.

## Activity 1.1               *Decision-making*

The questions in this activity are intended to help you to uncover different aspects of decision-making with reference to the case study.

1. What were the different decisions that Roger made in the case study?
2. What sources of information did Roger use to base his decisions on?

*continued overleaf . . .*

*continued . . .*

3. In what way was Roger's driving style adapted to the road conditions?
4. What could Roger have done differently to avoid having an accident?
5. What might the lorry driver have done to help prevent the accident?
6. Do you think the trip itself was really necessary or not? Why?
7. How successful were the outcomes of Roger's decision-making?
8. In what way might Roger be held accountable for what happened?

*Some possible answers can be found at the end of the chapter.*

The case study and Activity 1.1 help us to piece together key characteristics of decision-making.

- Decision-making applies judgement regarding our reasons for doing or not doing things.
- We use different information sources to support our judgement and decision-making.
- It involves choices about what, when, where, why and how we do things, and with or for whom.
- Evaluating decision-making involves assessing the choices made and their effectiveness.
- Decisions can be planned, unplanned or an urgent reaction to an emergency situation.
- We are always making different types of decisions, often without realising that we are.
- Freedom to make decisions is balanced by **accountability** in having to answer for them.

The style of the Transforming Nursing Practice series of books (to which this book belongs) is well suited to exploring decision-making because the books encourage learning through participation, thereby linking theory to practice. Similarly, clinical decision-making is the means by which we relate **theory** and research to practice in carrying out nursing care for our patients. This chapter begins by clarifying what we mean by clinical judgement and decision-making in nursing. We will briefly look at the development of nursing as a profession and how this impacts on our clinical decision-making. The structure of the book is then explained with reference to a research study on nursing students' development of clinical decision-making skills (Standing, 2005), followed by a summary. More case studies and learning activities are used to engage you in the process.

# What is clinical judgement and decision-making?

Nursing, like driving a car, involves carefully planned decisions (care plans), reacting to changing circumstances with unplanned decision-making (a patient looks upset so you check out why) and life-saving decisions in emergency situations (patient is choking so clear airway). In the last ten years clinical judgement and decision-making have been acknowledged as key processes in nursing. For example, the Royal College of Nursing (RCN) states that:

> *Nursing is the use of clinical judgement in the provision of care to enable people to improve, maintain, or recover health, to cope with health problems, and to achieve the best possible quality of life whatever their disease or disability, until death.*
> (RCN, 2003, p3)

This indicates that a nurse's ability to promote health, prevent illness, relieve suffering and give patients high quality care is dependent on applying effective clinical judgement. For the purposes of this book the following understanding of this important process applies:

> *Clinical judgement is informed opinion (using intuition, reflection and critical thinking) that relates observation and assessment of patients to identifying and evaluating alternative nursing options.*

Hence, clinical judgement involves reviewing the potential consequences (risks and benefits) of possible alternative actions before committing oneself one way or the other (decision-making). A judge also 'passes judgement', which is, in effect, a decision regarding the innocence or guilt of someone and the nature of any punishment for crimes committed. We are not judges; we are nurses. We do not want to get confused by mixing the two terms up. For us, judgement is not decision-making but it is closely related. It is used to review options before a decision is made.

The RCN's definition of nursing would benefit from adding decision-making. Decision-making links judgement to practice by acting on it in choosing from the available options. We are also accountable for the quality, safety and effectiveness of our clinical decision-making, as follows:

> *The nurse is a safe, caring and competent decision maker willing to accept personal and professional accountability for his/her actions and continuous learning. The nurse practises within a statutory framework and code of ethics delivering nursing practice (care) that is appropriately based on research, evidence and critical thinking that effectively responds to the needs of individual clients (patients) and diverse populations.*
>
> (Gonzalez and Wagenaar, 2003, cited in NMC, 2010a, p6)

The above definition includes decision-making, accountability and research evidence, but while it mentions **critical thinking**, it leaves out intuitive and reflective aspects of clinical judgement. This makes it favour a more scientific interpretation of evidence-based clinical decision making. A more inclusive interpretation of clinical judgement offers nurses greater flexibility in matching different types of **evidence** to the variable nature of clinical demands, as indicated in Figure 1.1.

*Figure 1.1: Matching different types of clinical judgement to time for decision-making*
Source: Adapted from Standing, 2005

Figure 1.1 shows that where there is no time to make decisions (such as an emergency situation, as when Roger avoided the lorry) we rely more on intuitive judgement. When we have time to access and evaluate relevant research, we rely more on a critical review of evidence (a more accurate weather forecast than that in the case study). The conscious application of critical thinking skills is gradually increased in reflective, patient and peer-aided, and system-aided (approved procedures) clinical judgement. We will look in detail at the impact of the various types of judgement in clinical decision-making in the remaining chapters of the book. Before concluding this section we need to agree a definition of clinical decision-making for nurses that incorporates clinical judgement (as defined earlier), evidence and accountability for our actions.

*Clinical decision-making applies clinical judgement to select the best possible evidence-based option to control risks and address patients' needs in high quality care for which you are accountable.*

Activity 1.2 gives you a chance to clarify your understanding of the terminology.

---

**Activity 1.2**          *Reflection*

Think about what has been said in this section and answer the following questions as best you can.

1. What are the similarities and differences between clinical judgement and decision-making?
2. What are the benefits of good clinical judgement and decision-making skills in nursing?
3. How would you describe critical thinking skills and why are they so important in nursing?

*Some possible answers can be found at the end of the chapter.*

---

You should now be clearer about what these terms mean, and ready to look at how they relate to the development of nursing as a profession and the key concepts associated with it.

# Development of nursing, key concepts and clinical decision-making

Developing our decision-making ability is not a substitute for learning about the wide range of knowledge, skills and attitudes used in nursing. Key concepts of humans, environment, health and nursing (Fawcett, 2005) are adapted to structure Table 1.1, which summarises 150 years of professional development and its impact on our roles, clinical judgement and decision-making.

The idea of condensing and presenting you with a 150-year 'potted history' of nursing in Table 1.1 is not to press a panic button about names, dates and theories that you might be unfamiliar with – you are not expected to memorise it. It is something that offers a coherent overview of the key concepts and principles of nursing, the diverse scope of our roles as nurses, and the range of information sources and processes used in our clinical judgement and decision-making.

| Concepts | Meanings of, interaction between, and relevance of concepts |
|---|---|
| Human being | • Shaped by nature (genetically predetermined traits) and nurture (constant interaction physically, psychologically and socially with the environment).<br>• Range of biological, psychological, social, philosophical and spiritual needs.<br>• Developmental milestones during lifespan: from birth – dependent child, adolescent, creative independent adult, less independent old age – to death.<br>• Basic human rights to life, self-determination, freedom from oppression.<br>• Self-care ability: resist infection, recover from injury/illness, adapt to disability. |
| Environment | • Physical: air, food, water, warmth, shelter, natural resources to support life.<br>• Social: family, culture, politics/economics/law, education, religion, technology. |
| Health | • *Physical, mental and social well being and not merely the absence of disease or infirmity* (WHO, 1948); product of interaction between human beings and environment to address their needs (health) or not to (ill health); variations between cultures in how health and ill health are interpreted. |
| Nurse's role and decision making | • Human advocacy: enable people to adopt healthy lifestyle, prevent ill health, recover from illness or injury, adapt to disability, and have a peaceful death.<br>• Nursing theories' view of role: keep environment clean to promote healing (Nightingale, 1860); help people to address bio–psycho–social–spiritual needs or activities of living (Henderson, 1966; Roper et al., 2000); use interpersonal relationship, therapeutic communication and cultural sensitivity in enabling people to cope with stress, enhance mental health and find meaning in their lives (Peplau, 1952; Leininger, 1985; Parse, 1992); encourage holistic (bio-psycho-social) self-care or adaptation by tailoring interventions according to a person's level of dependence or independence (Orem, 1980; Roy, 1980); apply principles of human caring to achieve all of the above (Watson, 1988).<br>• Clinical decision-making in nursing is informed by: systematic problem solving (Yura and Walsh, 1973); reflective practice (Schön, 1983); expert intuitive judgement (Benner, 1984); and accessing, evaluating and applying research in evidence-based practice (Fleming and Fenton, 2002; Ellis, 2010) |

*Table 1.1: Key concepts in nursing: relevance to nurses' role and decision-making*

# Human beings

You have no doubt heard of the terms **person-centred**, client-centred and **patient-centred care**, but are you sure what they mean? The concept human being (Table 1.1) offers a way to make sense of the above 'buzz words'. For example, our uniqueness as individuals is both genetically and environmentally determined, and this will manifest itself in our physical and psychological characteristics, variations in social behaviour, and self-care ability. Despite our differences we are all entitled to have our human rights protected during healthcare. This is explored in more depth in Chapter 2 (Collaborative clinical decision-making), and Chapter 9 (Ethical sensitivity in decision-making).

# Environment and health

The concepts of environment and health prompt us to reflect on the ways that cultural values affect an individual's health, as the following case study illustrates.

## Case study

*In 2008, an 11-year-old girl died when she went into a diabetic coma and stopped breathing at her home in a rural 'white' community in the USA. She developed symptoms of diabetes (thirst, weight loss, tiredness, frequency of urination) one month before, but her parents decided not to take her to the doctor because they believed they could cure her through the power of prayer.*

The case study shows we cannot assume that everyone living in the same country shares the same cultural values or that there are no cultural differences within ethnic groups. The USA is one of the most scientifically and technologically advanced countries in the world and yet this appeared not to inform the rural community referred to. It is tragic that this young girl died when insulin could have saved her, but it will be even more tragic if we do not honour her life by learning something from her passing. One thing we can learn is that all of the knowledge and decision-making skills outlined in Table 1.1 did not help the girl because it was not accessible to her. We need, therefore, to provide 'culture congruent care' (Leininger, 1985) so that such families will not be prevented from making use of health services that could prolong their lives by fear that we will not respect their values. There is a second learning point here: if we do not keep up to date with developments in research and nursing knowledge, we will be behaving in a similar way to the girl's parents, except that we will be placing many more lives in jeopardy.

# Nursing

The concept of nursing in Table 1.1 reminds us that our first duty is to champion the health and well-being of our patients. The overview of theories conveys the breadth and depth of holistic (bio-psycho-socio-spiritual) knowledge associated with nursing, applicable to all the pathways. Collectively, they support patient-centred, interpersonally skilled, holistic, systematic, critical, reflective, health-promoting, evidence-based, culturally sensitive and caring nursing. These attributes are also found in the standards for pre-registration nursing education (NMC, 2010).

According to Snyder (1995) *The theoretical or conceptual model used by a nurse provides the basis for making complex decisions that are crucial in the delivery of good nursing care* (p33). However, when the RCN surveyed nurses about their understanding of nursing (in compiling a definition), they discovered that many nurses found it hard to describe their knowledge or skills. Similarly, Clark (2006) reported that nurses often *find it difficult to put into words the concept of nursing that they hold inside their heads* (p33). For theory to enhance practice it must be accessible, understandable, relevant and applicable. If the language used to explain ideas is complicated or confusing, then even if it contains useful information, it will not be understood. A **theory–practice gap** occurs where the formal learning of **espoused theories** in universities is in conflict with informal, work-based **theories-in-use** in professional practice (Argyris and Schön, 1974). Activity 1.3 asks you to explore any experience you have of a 'theory–practice gap'.

---

### Activity 1.3          *Evidence-based practice*

This activity is intended to help you to identify what has helped to guide your clinical practice and to identify discrepancies between taught theory and what actually happens in clinical practice.

- Identify and describe something you learned at university that you applied in practice, and explain what difference it made to the way you worked, and what the outcome was.
- Identify and describe something you learned at university that you found difficult to apply in practice and explain why this was so.
- Identify and describe something you learned and applied in clinical practice and explain what difference it made to the way you worked, and what the outcome was.
- Identify and describe any examples of conflicting information and advice about nursing care regarding university 'espoused' theory and clinical practice 'theories-in-use'.

*Discuss your responses with colleagues, mentors or personal tutors. As this is for your own reflection, no answer is given at the end of the chapter.*

---

Activity 1.3 recognises that you may experience differences between theory and research input at university, and the customs and practices developed in clinical areas. It also encourages us to appreciate the positive contribution both can potentially make to our development in clinical decision-making skills. As stated in the introduction, clinical decision-making involves theory applied to practice, and it is important that we are able to explain reasons for nursing actions. If we are unable to, how can we enable patients to give informed consent to treatment and care?

The final subsection of 'nursing' in Table 1.1 describes the emergence of a range of clinical decision-making styles associated with different types of clinical judgement and levels of critical thinking (see also Figure 1.1). Intuitive judgement is valuable when decisions have to be made quickly, but as it tends to function at a subconscious level, it is often difficult to clearly articulate reasons for decisions. Critical review and application of research-based evidence is valuable when there is time to plan care thoroughly, and as it is a conscious process of judgement and decision-making, it is open to scrutiny by others. This enables the communication of nursing knowledge and skills, and greater public accountability for decision-making, which are important because:

- nurses need to consult, negotiate, discuss and explain the reasons for their proposed practical care to patients, families, other nurses and members of the healthcare team;
- nurses need to keep clear written records as evidence of the care they have provided;
- each nurse is accountable for the quality of care (its safety and effectiveness) that they give to patients, and must be able to justify and defend their actions if challenged to do so.

Figure 1.2 links developments in nursing to four vital characteristics of safe and effective clinical judgement and decision-making: practicality, logic, relevance and rigour (Standing and Standing, 2010).

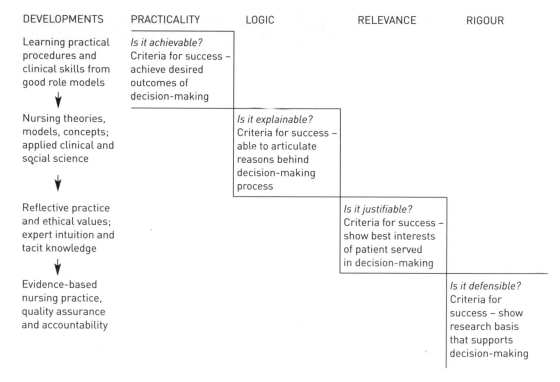

*Figure 1.2: Developments in nursing in relation to four vital decision-making criteria*

Figure 1.2 shows four stages in the development of nursing as a profession (from learning practical procedures to **evidence-based practice**), cross referenced to corresponding, vital clinical decision-making criteria (from practicality to rigour). In other words, each stage of our historical development is associated with a particular strength in relation to clinical judgement and decision-making (e.g. nursing theories – logic; reflective practice – relevance). For our clinical judgement and decision-making to be of the highest quality we need to apply all four criteria (practicality, logic, relevance and rigour). This means we need to incorporate all the knowledge, skills, attitudes and values attributed to the stages of nursing's development (practical procedures, nursing theories, reflective practice and evidence-based practice). Due to its unique structure, this book is going to help you to achieve this.

# The book's unique structure: ten types of clinical decision-making

## The research study

The book's structure is shaped by a unique research study (using **hermeneutic phenomenology**) exploring nursing students' experiences of clinical decision-making on a four-year developmental journey in becoming and practising as registered nurses (Standing, 2005).

Twenty students kept reflective journals of their experiences in acquiring and applying clinical decision-making skills throughout the pre-registration programme and first year as staff nurses (Adult/Mental Health/Child) between 2000 and 2004. This was supplemented by four tape-recorded in-depth interviews with each student (at 3–5, 18–20, 32–34 and 42–48 months). The interviews helped students to recall and discuss critical incidents they had experienced and to clarify their personal conceptions (understanding) of nursing, and their perceptions of clinical decision-making skills. This generated 250,000 words of interview transcripts, which were thematically analysed, revealing a total of ten conceptions of nursing and ten perceptions of clinical decision-making. The themes were checked with the students, and developed and refined as necessary to accurately reflect their views, and to summarise their experiences.

A 'matrix model' was created by cross-referencing nursing conceptions/clinical decision-making types (Standing, 2005, 2007, 2010). It helps nurses to integrate key concepts, skills, attitudes and values with the clinical decision-making criteria in Table 1.1 and Figure 1.2. Table 1.2 lists the conceptions of nursing and perceptions of clinical decision-making. Each of the remaining chapters in the book is dedicated to a detailed exploration of one of the decision-making types, which are also cross-referenced against all ten of the identified conceptions of nursing.

| Conceptions of nursing | Types of clinical decision-making |
|---|---|
| Caring | Collaborative |
| Listening and being there | Observation |
| Practical procedures | Systematic |
| Knowledge and understanding | Standardised |
| Communicating | Prioritising |
| Patience | Experience and intuition |
| Teamwork | Reflective |
| Paperwork and electronic record | Ethical sensitivity |
| Empathising and non-judgemental | Accountability |
| Professional | Confidence |

*Table 1.2 Nurses' understanding of nursing and clinical decision-making skills*

The themes in Table 1.2 summarise students' personal, practical and theoretical understanding of clinical decision-making, and support the view that *Professional practice requires knowledge derived from research and theory, from professional practice, and from personal experience* (Higgs and Titchen, 2001, pp4–5). The themes complement the nursing theories referred to earlier and standards for pre-registration nursing education (NMC, 2010a).

# Applying ten types of decision-making

Before we look at each of the decision-making types in detail in Chapters 2–11, the following case study applies all ten types, to give you a flavour of the book as a whole. It shows that if a nursing student is observant, they can make a real positive difference to a vulnerable person's life and complement the role of an experienced nurse and healthcare team.

## Case study: Frightened to use the lift

*Pearl is a second-year nursing student on placement in a community health centre. She goes with Shirley, a district nurse, to take a blood sample from Maude, aged 73, who is unable to get out much due to her arthritis. Maude's mobility is also hampered because she lives on the eighteenth floor of a high-rise block of flats (owned by the local council). While Shirley is attending to Maude, Pearl talks to her daughter Beth, aged 32, who has Down's syndrome (a genetic abnormality that used to be called mongolism and is associated with intellectual disability and unusual appearance – flat face, slanting eyes, small mouth, and sometimes protruding tongue and fingers with webbed skin). Beth asks Pearl if she would like a cup of tea, adding that the people in the church hall, where she volunteers, always say she makes a lovely cup of tea. Pearl, seeing that Beth's hands are blistered, says 'Not at the moment, thank you' and asks 'What happened to your hands?' Beth's demeanour changes from cheerful to serious and sad. She tells Pearl that since she has been doing all the shopping, a nasty family on the seventh floor call her horrible names if they see her in the lift. She has asked them to stop it but they just do it more. So for the last six months Beth has only used the lift between the eighth and eighteenth floors. She walks up and down seven flights of stairs between the ground floor and the eighth floor to avoid seeing the 'nasty' family and has blisters from pulling the fully laden trolley up the stairs. Pearl says she is sorry to hear that she is being bullied and asks if Beth has told her mum about what has happened. Beth says she hasn't because it is her job to look after her mum now.*

*Pearl reports this to Shirley, who praises Beth for doing such a great job of looking after her mum but adds that she must also look after herself. Keeping the bullying a secret will not make it stop, and if she falls down the stairs, nobody will know she is there. They agree a plan for Shirley to inform the GP, Council, social services and police so that the offending family are made to stop bullying Beth. Although Maude loves the view from her flat, she agrees that it might also be time to ask the council for more suitable accommodation nearer the ground. In the meantime, Beth will arrange to go shopping with a friendly neighbour so that she feels safe using the lift all the way from ground to the eighteenth floor. Beth asks Pearl how to send texts on the mobile phone her mum ordered for her, and Pearl shows her this and also how to store numbers. Beth is happy that she can now text her friends. Shirley tells Pearl that she did a really good job in finding out about Beth being bullied.*

The case study brings into perspective the key concepts outlined in Table 1.1. Beth's rights as a human being had been violated just because she looked different from other people. Problems getting in and out of the block of flats highlight the way in which the physical and social environment can affect someone's health and well-being (too frightened to use the lift). With regard to her nursing skills, Pearl was caring, attentive and empathising, and she communicated with Beth in a way she felt comfortable with. She applied technical skills in showing Beth how to send texts on her mobile phone and demonstrated teamwork skills by informing Shirley about the bullying. The range of clinical decision-making types used by Shirley, Pearl and other agencies is summarised in Table 1.3. The main thrust of short-term decision-making was focused on safeguarding Beth by implementing legal sanctions to stop the offenders if necessary, and ensuring that Beth feels safe when she goes out stopping. Longer term, it is likely that Maude and Beth will be rehoused.

| Types | Examples of decision-making types used in the case study |
|---|---|
| *Collaborative* | Tell GP/Council Housing Officer/social services/police that Beth is being bullied. |
| *Observation* | Noticing Beth's hands were blistered and that it seemed to be worrying her. |
| *Systematic* | Authorities investigate – tell bullies to stop or face eviction and prosecution. |
| *Standardised* | Discrimination illegal (Equality Act 2010) and breaches tenancy agreement. |
| *Prioritising* | Stopping the bullying for Beth to use lift safely; review housing options. |
| *Experience and intuition* | Sensing Beth unhappy, identifying problem by enabling her to talk about it. |
| *Reflective* | Ask Beth to go out with a buddy she feels safe with; her neighbour agrees. |
| *Ethical sensitivity* | Respect Beth's right to come and go in the lift without fear of intimidation. |
| *Accountability* | Professional obligation to safeguard a vulnerable adult if abuse suspected. |
| *Confidence* | Enable Beth to send/read texts and store numbers on her mobile phone. |

*Table 1.3: Applying ten decision-making types to the case study*

The importance of decision-making in this case is graphically illustrated in Chapter 2 when a mother and daughter with intellectual disabilities are not given the support they deserve.

## Chapter summary

This chapter introduced you to clinical judgement and decision-making for nursing students. We began by clarifying what the terms meant and their similarities and differences. We noted that there is a range of clinical judgement from intuitive with less critical thinking to critical review of evidence with more critical thinking, and that these were related to fast emergency decision-making and slow, well-planned decision-making, respectively. We had a brief overview of the historical development of nursing as a profession regarding key concepts – human beings, environment, health and nursing. We saw how this can help us understand and explain nursing knowledge, skills, attitudes and values – for example, what patient-centred means. We skipped through a variety of nursing theories supporting a holistic understanding of people. We looked at various approaches to clinical decision-making in nursing, how each one has particular strengths and how combining them all seems sensible, and we looked at vital criteria – practicality, logic, relevance and rigour – to quality assure decision-making. Lastly, a research study was described that followed a group of students through the nursing programme and first year as staff nurses to explore how they identified, developed and applied clinical decision-making skills. Ten wide-ranging types of decision-making were identified from the research, which will be used as the basis for each of the remaining chapters in this book. They will be cross-referenced to conceptions of nursing identified in the research study (Standing, 2005) to promote integration of professional values in nurses' clinical decision-making. The final case study, 'Frightened to use the lift', showed how all ten decision-making types were used in caring for a vulnerable adult who had been victimised. It also enabled us to see how theoretical concepts (human beings, environment, health and nursing) are applied in practice. In Chapter 4 of this book we will see how these key concepts inform an 'activities of living' model (Roper et al., 2000) when nursing someone with a long-term medical condition. Each remaining chapter will therefore build on this one in developing your knowledge, skills, attitudes and values in clinical judgement and decision-making. I hope this chapter has whetted your appetite.

## Activities: brief outline answers

### Activity 1.1 Decision-making (page 6)

You may have included the following points.

1.  What were the different decisions that Roger made in the case study? To collect son from university; timing of trip; continuing despite snow; avoiding lorry.
2.  What sources of information did Roger use to base his decisions on? Looked at sky; heard weather forecast.
3.  In what way was Roger's driving style adapted to the road conditions? Kept within speed restriction; tried to slow down with gears to avoid skidding.
4.  What could Roger have done differently to avoid having an accident? Not gone; researched weather forecast; turned back when it snowed; kept longer distance from lorry in front; changed lane before so not behind lorry so could see road ahead.

5.  What might the lorry driver have done to help prevent the accident? Cleaned back of lorry to make brake lights visible; stayed on the inner lane.
6.  Do you think the trip itself was really necessary or not? Why? With hindsight risks outweighed benefits given surprising early snowfall.
7.  How successful were the outcomes of Roger's decision-making? Unsuccessful: failed to pick up son, car was a write off, hit/got hit by other cars. Successful: avoided more serious injury by avoiding driving into the back of the lorry.
8.  In what way might Roger be held accountable for what happened? Police checked if anyone was to blame but concluded 'no'; telling son he cannot make it; may lose no claims bonus; vehicle he hit may claim off his insurance.

## Activity 1.2 Reflection (page 8)

You may have included the following points:

1.  *Similarities* – both are used to define nursing; apply critical thinking; consider alternative options; apply theory to practice.
    *Differences* – one assesses options, the other chooses and implements one of the options.
2.  *Benefits* – high quality evidence-based nursing that addresses patients' healthcare needs.
3.  *Description* – questioning assumptions of self and others, addressing gaps in knowledge needed to achieve aims, challenging illogical beliefs, evaluating adequacy of research evidence, presenting a logical, evidence-based argument and defending it when challenged
    *Importance* – without it, you cannot achieve the above benefits; registered nurses are accountable and have to justify their actions when challenged.

## Further reading

**Ellis, P** (2010) *Evidence-based Practice in Nursing.* Exeter: Learning Matters.

A good introduction to a wide range of evidence used to inform clinical judgement and decisions.

**Hall, C and Ritchie, D** (2009) *What is Nursing?* Exeter: Learning Matters.

Helpful overview of the theory and practice of nursing.

**Mckenna, P and Slevin, D** (2008) *Nursing Models, Theories and Practice.* Oxford: Blackwell Publishing.

A useful exploration of nursing models and theories, which raises interesting questions about whether and how they are used in practice.

**Williamson, GR, Jenkinson, T and Proctor-Childs, T** (2010) *Contexts of Contemporary Nursing.* Exeter: Learning Matters.

Informative account of developments in healthcare and their impact on nurses' responsibilities.

## Useful websites

**www.nursingtheory.net/gt_alm.html**

This website has helpful summaries of most theories/models and useful links to some theorists' websites.

**Mencap.org.uk**

Website of the learning disabilities charity. Very informative and supportive with lots of interesting video clips.

# Chapter 2
## Collaborative clinical decision-making

*continued . . .*

*By the second progression point:*

vi.   Forms appropriate and constructive professional relationships with families and other carers.

6.  People can trust the newly registered nurse to engage therapeutically and actively listen to their needs and concerns, responding using skills that are helpful, providing information that is clear, accurate, meaningful and free from jargon.

    *By the first progression point:*

    v.   Effectively communicates people's stated needs and wishes to other professionals.

## Cluster: Organisational aspects of care

11. People can trust the newly registered graduate nurse to safeguard children and adults from vulnerable situations and support and protect them from harm.

    *By the first progression point:*

    ii.   Shares information with colleagues and seeks advice from appropriate sources where there is a concern or uncertainty.

    *By entry to the register:*

    viii. Works collaboratively with other agencies to develop, implement and monitor strategies to safeguard and protect individuals and groups who are in vulnerable situations.

12. People can trust the newly registered graduate nurse to respond to their feedback and a wide range of other sources to learn, develop and improve services.

    *By the second progression point:*

    iv.   Takes feedback from colleagues, managers and other departments seriously and shares the messages and learning with other members of the team.

## Chapter aims

By the end of this chapter, you should be able to:

*   explain what collaborative clinical decision-making means;
*   give examples of collaborative decision-making with patients;
*   describe collaborative decision-making within the healthcare team;
*   understand your role in collaborating with healthcare team members;
*   appreciate that collaboration is vital for integrated patient-centred care.

# Introduction

This, and remaining chapters of the book, each explore a different clinical decision-making theme identified when researching nursing students' experience and perceptions of their developmental journey in becoming (and practising as) registered nurses (Standing, 2005). Of the ten themes identified in the research we begin with **collaborative decision-making**.

1. Collaborating with patients and others lies at the heart of good nursing practice.
2. There was more agreement about the importance of collaborative decision-making by nurses in the research study than about any of the other themes they identified.
3. This and subsequent chapters will help you to participate in a collaborative way by testing out ideas presented and relating them to your experience.

This suggests that collaboration is central not only to nursing practice and management but also to nursing research and education. Collaborative decision-making, therefore, seems a logical starting point on our journey in exploring nurses' clinical decision-making skills together.

The chapter begins by asking 'What is collaborative decision-making?' and looking at the similarities and differences between collaboration, co-operation, consultation, negotiation and collusion. These issues are then related to our professional context by asking 'What is collaborative clinical decision-making in nursing?' The rest of the chapter is dedicated to applying collaborative clinical decision-making in nursing when working with patients and families, with other healthcare professionals, and when integrating working with patients/families and other health professionals to give high quality care. Practical examples and case studies illustrate applications of collaborative decision-making in different clinical contexts. Various activities encourage you to relate chapter contents to your own personal and clinical experience. Finally, the strengths and weaknesses of collaborative clinical decision-making are summarised.

# What is collaborative decision-making?

Collaborative decisions are joint decisions between two or more people for the purpose of achieving an agreed aim. For example, as a result of the May 2010 general election in the United Kingdom (UK), a coalition government was formed by the Conservatives and Liberal Democrats. Despite their different political values, the two parties agreed to work together to govern the country and reduce the national debt with a cost-cutting economic policy. Collaboration, therefore, involves:

- consultation to express opinions about what needs to be done;
- negotiation to identify a solution with which all parties can agree;
- co-operation to suspend differences and work towards shared aims.

Individually, these processes represent only one aspect of collaboration; but collectively they describe key principles of collaborative decision-making. Enabling everyone to have their say has limited purpose if their views are ignored when decisions are being made. Plans to tackle problems are limited if they are not implemented as agreed. A commitment to working together is limited if 'not rocking the boat' inhibits debate or cultivates compliance to the most dominant view. Hence, combining and balancing consultation, negotiation and co-operation are essential to enable effective discussion, agreement and joint action in collaborative decision-making.

## Activity 2.1 — *Decision-making*

Describe your involvement in collaborative decisions outside nursing – for example, what to cook, what film to watch, where to go on holiday, going shopping, etc. Identify what you had in common with those with whom you agreed decisions, and the aims you think you shared. Reflect on how easy or difficult it was to agree what to do, what each person's contribution to the process was, and how successful you think the outcome was for all those concerned.

- What are the key features of collaborative decision-making that your examples illustrate?

*Some possible answers are included at the end of the chapter.*

The word 'collaboration' can have negative associations. For example, a 'collaborator' during the Second World War was regarded as a traitor working with the enemy. Negative forms of collaboration involve collusion where prevailing social, political or moral values are undermined by a shared, more secretive alternative agenda. This results in inconsistency between what you say publicly you believe in and what you actually believe in and do 'behind the scenes'. Some examples are given below.

- Hard-line Conservatives and Liberal Democrats might feel their parties were colluding by 'selling out' their respective core values in joining together to gain political power.
- The coalition government's justification for reducing incapacity benefit claims was that the system is abused, and if they do not take action, they collude with those being unfairly rewarded.
- If a nurse says nothing when a colleague forgets to wash their hands before attending to patients, then the nurse is colluding with the colleague in endangering patients' health and safety (in this case the stated values of promoting health are undermined by a lack of assertiveness).

Activity 2.2 provides an opportunity for you to identify instances of collusion you might have come across.

## Activity 2.2 — *Reflection*

See if you can recall any examples of collusion from what you have observed or experienced. Briefly describe the circumstances, and why you think those involved colluded with each other. This could be during your nursing programme, in clinical practice, or in non-nursing contexts.

- How does your example illustrate the characteristics of collusion described above?

*Some possible answers are included at the end of the chapter.*

We will look in more detail at potential risks and consequences of collusion later in the chapter.

Positive forms of collaborative decision-making are part of sustaining productive relationships in all aspects of human interaction (including healthcare), as illustrated in the case study below.

## Case study: Give and take in relationships

*At the beginning of their nursing programme, students were asked about their understanding and experience of decision-making. Jo talked about making joint decisions with her fiancé:*

*'Decision-making between the two of us is a 50–50 thing unless one has particularly strong views and the other hasn't. If we've both got strong views, then it's "telly off" and we have a debate about it. When it comes to life decisions, he wants to join the fire brigade and I have been considering a nursing career in the army. We agreed to see whether he gets into the fire brigade. If he does, I can put off the army for a few years as I can be a nurse in the NHS or the army but he can only be a fireman in the fire brigade. It's very much "give and take"; I'll compromise or he'll compromise depending on what's more important and who can still be happy. I'll probably be happy working in an NHS A and E department or in an army field hospital in Afghanistan.'*

The case study is an example of collaborative decision-making because it involves more than one person, the respective parties each make a distinct contribution, and they work together to achieve a common aim. The aim in this instance is to enable the couple to maintain a sustainable partnership while realising their respective career ambitions, in a way that both are happy with. It involves listening to and respecting each person's opinions (consultation), flexibility to compromise where priorities may clash (negotiation), and good will in deferring some of one's own preferences, where necessary, to support others in achieving their goals (co-operation).

## Activity 2.3                                                            *Decision-making*

Identify a joint (collaborative) nursing decision that you were involved in or witnessed, and briefly describe who was involved, their respective contributions (including yours), the shared aim you were all hoping to achieve, the agreed decision, the action taken and the resulting outcome. Try to identify examples of:

*   consultation – how each person's opinions were taken on board;
*   negotiation – how agreement was reached about main priorities;
*   co-operation – how behaviour was adjusted to achieve goals.

*As this is to help you relate collaborative decision-making to your own experience, there is no specimen answer provided.*

Having identified and reflected on key aspects of collaborative decision-making, we can now look in more detail at how this relates to the clinical decisions in which nurses participate.

# What is collaborative clinical decision-making in nursing?

Before we can answer this fully we need to recap what we mean by the term 'clinical decision-making' in nursing, which was explored in Chapter 1, and is summarised as follows:

> *Clinical decision-making in nursing involves applying critical thinking skills to select the best available evidence-based option to control risks and address patients' needs in the provision of high quality care that nurses are accountable for.*

We also need to recap what is meant by the term 'nursing'. This is necessary to identify who might be involved in collaborative decisions, knowing what the purpose is, and how respective roles are negotiated to work together in achieving agreed goals. For the purposes of this book, nursing theory and definitions (Gonzalez and Wagenaar, 2003; RCN, 2003) referred to in Chapter 1 are used to create the following working definition of nursing:

> *Nursing promotes health, recovery from illness or injury, adaptation to disability, and dignity when facing death, in patient-centred care applying bio–psycho–social–spiritual knowledge, skills and ethical values to ensure safe and effective clinical judgement and decision-making and high quality evidence-based practice.*

The patient-centred focus reinforces the importance of collaborating with patients and relatives. The broad scope of nursing activities (from promoting health to enabling a dignified death) also requires collaboration with other health professionals who have specialist skills to help identify or address patients' wide-ranging needs. The aim we all share is to promote or restore health and relieve suffering in giving high quality care that is relevant to patients' healthcare needs.

We cannot, therefore, give patient-centred nursing care without collaborating with patients and others. Being patient-centred involves: consulting with patients to identify their preferences and get feedback about their care; explaining options, giving information to help them decide if they consent to proposed treatments; negotiating and implementing action plans that are relevant and responsive to patients' unique needs; and co-operating with other healthcare professionals by working together as a team to achieve this. By putting together our understanding of nursing, decision-making and collaboration, we arrive at a definition for the purposes of this book:

> *Collaborative clinical decision-making in nursing involves consulting, negotiating and co-operating with patients, relatives, nurses, mentors, managers, health professionals and other relevant agencies, to promote health and to inform the delivery of high quality patient-centred care that is relevant to their specific needs.*

Each stage of good patient-centred nursing care requires collaborative decision-making with patients and families (sometimes referred to as service users and carers in public documents relating to healthcare). It often involves inter-professional or inter-agency teamwork. Before moving on to explore this in more depth, Activity 2.4 asks you to 'pause for thought' regarding the relevance of collaborative decision-making in the context of evidence-based practice.

## Activity 2.4                                                        *Critical thinking*

This activity is to help you to apply critical thinking skills (which are an important feature of effective clinical judgement and decision-making). Critical thinking involves using logical reasoning to question assumptions or inconsistencies in beliefs, arguments, available evidence and clinical practice, and to explain, justify and defend our decisions and actions. The descriptions of clinical decision-making and the nursing profession given above both mention being evidence-based. It was also argued that collaborative clinical decision-making is vital in high quality nursing care. If this is so, then logically collaborative decisions must in some way contribute to evidence-based practice in nursing. Please take a moment to think about this, and then use your critical thinking skills to work out a possible answer to the following question:

• How can collaborative clinical decision-making contribute to evidence-based nursing?

*Some possible answers are included at the end of the chapter.*

If you need further help in completing Activity 2.4, you may find another book in this series, *Evidence-based Practice in Nursing* (Ellis, 2010), useful. Chapter 1 has a model that includes patient preferences and views of other professionals as information sources that influence the delivery of patient-centred care.

Now that we have got to grips with the meaning of collaborative clinical decision-making in nursing, we are ready to explore different ways it can be effectively applied to practice.

# Applying collaborative clinical decision-making in nursing

The application of collaborative clinical decision-making is an essential part of nurse–patient relationships and inter-professional teamwork in hospital and community health, or social care settings. We start off by looking at collaborating with patients and families, followed by inter-professional collaboration, and then how to integrate the two strands in collaborative healthcare.

## Collaborating with patients and families

Collaborative clinical decision-making is dependent on establishing effective relationships with patients and families. However, learning how to communicate and consult with patients, in order to find out what their opinions and preferences are, can take a while to achieve, as illustrated in the following case study.

## Case study: Conversations with patients

*Connie is a nursing student nearing the end of her first year. She reflects on how she learnt to focus more on patients' needs during her conversations with them:*

*'I realise that I like talking to people. People that have been sitting in a hospital bed are bored and they often want to talk. There was an elderly lady that I took a "shine" to. I know you're not supposed to. I spent more time with her because she was more talkative than other people and I found it easy to think of things to say to her. Then I suddenly realised that she probably wasn't interested in what I was saying, and that it was she who really needed someone to talk to. I thought to myself "I will just let her do the talking", and since then, I have been able to stop myself from "rambling away" with patients and been more attentive to what they might need.'*

Connie became aware that her interest in talking to a patient reflected her personal needs rather than the patient's. This increased level of self-awareness enabled her to listen more and say less, in order to help patients talk about issues affecting them. In doing so, Connie indicated that she had translated her social conversation skills into purposeful, professional and patient-centred communication/interpersonal skills that increased her effectiveness in consulting with patients.

In Activity 2.5 you are asked to think about your own experience of communicating with patients.

## Activity 2.5                                               *Communication*

Think about and describe an experience in communicating with patients. Like Connie, you may find some patients easier and more interesting to talk to than others. Why do you think it is vital to have a good relationship and be skilled at consulting with *all* patients in eliciting their views?

*Some possible answers are included at the end of the chapter.*

Connie experienced a tension between using social conversation skills to establish relationships with patients and developing other therapeutic communication skills that focus more directly on addressing patients' concerns. Contact with patients provides continuous experiential learning opportunities to refine our communication skills while physically, emotionally and psychologically engaged in interpersonal therapeutic activities. In this way we learn to blend personal, practical and professional qualities in shaping our nursing identities and roles (Higgs and Titchen, 2001). We will be looking at this in more detail in Chapter 7, Experience and intuition in decision-making, and in Chapter 8, Reflective judgement and decision-making. Theoretical approaches can also help to inform nurses' understanding, development, application and validation of their communication and interpersonal skills (Bach and Grant, 2009). Without this ability to 'tune in' to what patients' healthcare concerns are, whether in hospital or at home, collaborative clinical decision-making with them is not really possible. It is not surprising, then, that communication skills feature strongly in the NMC Code when collaborative person-centred care is described:

*Collaborate with those in your care*
- *You must listen to the people in your care and respond to their concerns and preferences.*
- *You must support people in caring for themselves to improve and maintain their health.*
- *You must recognise and respect the contribution that people make to their own care and wellbeing.*
- *You must make arrangements to meet people's language and communication needs.*
- *You must share with people, in a way they can understand, the information they want or need to know about their health.*

(NMC, 2008, p3)

These requirements are also reflected in various Standards (and Essential Skills Clusters) for Pre-Registration Nursing Education (NMC, 2010a), as revealed at the start of this chapter.

# Building on collaboration

Knowing that developing and maintaining a good nurse–patient relationship is an important factor in providing high quality care and enabling effective collaborative clinical decision-making does not guarantee it always happens in practice. Many areas of nursing are highly pressurised, and this can sometimes result in less consultation with patients about their preferences, less time to negotiate with them about what their contribution might be to the care process, and greater expectation that patients should simply co-operate with prescribed treatments. In the following case study one nurse finds a way to incorporate more consultation with patients in a busy ward.

## Case study: Introducing a way to collaborate with patients

*Serena is a second year nursing student on placement in a surgical ward. In reflecting on her experience she describes how a great deal of pre- and post-operative nursing care has involved carefully following standardised procedures in a predominantly medical model of care. She feels it has encouraged a task-orientated approach to ensure that vital observations of patients and procedures are carried out, and that this can distract nurses from providing patient-centred care.*

*Serena noted that after patients had lunch, the nurses usually sat down to update individualised care plans for those for whom they were responsible. Serena says, 'I like to go round the beds to ask each person if there is anything they would like me to include in their records about how they are progressing and about any concerns or preferences they might have; and by listening and looking at each person I get a mental picture of how they are feeling and what care they might need.'*

In the ward where Serena was working, it was not customary practice for nurses to check with each patient before writing up the notes. Many were happy to take the weight off their feet after a busy morning, and recording their observations and activities provided an opportunity for this (once patients' most pressing needs had been addressed). Serena used her initiative by inviting patients' contribution in updating their care plans as it gave her an opportunity to interact with them, which she liked, it enabled her to observe or assess them more closely, and she felt it was important they were involved in discussing the care they had received and plans for continuing care.

Leadership and management styles determine the policies, customs and practices of nurses in clinical areas. This activity invites you to think about the implications of the case study regarding the management of change in adopting collaborative practices to enhance patient-centred care.

Please take a moment to reflect on your own clinical experience and see whether you can relate to any of the issues referred to by Serena.

- If you were a patient, would you like or dislike a nurse coming to ask you what you think about your care following your lunch? Why?
- If you were a nursing colleague of Serena, do you think you would praise or criticise her actions? Why?
- What might be obstacles to collaborative decision-making and patient-centred care?

*Some possible answers to the last question are included at the end of the chapter.*

Introducing and sustaining practice changes to overcome obstacles to greater collaborative decision-making and patient-centred care need effective leadership and management. Serena felt well supported by her mentor, who admired her energy and commitment to patients and demonstrated this by emulating the way Serena consulted patients in updating their records. The ward manager also commented on the good quality of Serena's nursing notes during team meetings. This encouraged other nurses to follow suit, which they found rewarding as most of the patients appreciated feeling more involved in their own care. In terms of change theory, Serena was an adventurous innovator who took a risk in trying out a new way to update notes that involved collaborating with patients. The mentor and ward sister were 'early adopters' who exercised leadership in supporting Serena's actions and encouraging others to try it out for themselves. Nurses might adopt the change fairly quickly ('early majority'), after a longer period of deliberation ('late majority'), or eventually when the change seems inevitable ('laggards') (Rogers, 1962). Barriers to change, such as lack of incentive (NICE, 2007a), were reduced through the mentor's and ward manager's flexible and responsive leadership, and by the nurses gaining a sense of satisfaction from adapting and developing their clinical practice.

Even in areas such as mental health care where, traditionally, more attention has been focused on what patients are thinking and feeling, and enabling patients to develop ways of dealing with various stressors, effective collaborative clinical decision-making can be difficult to achieve. The case study below demonstrates this, while reinforcing the benefit of having a supportive mentor.

## Case study: Preventing a psychotic relapse

*Franco is a third-year student on placement with a community mental health team. One of his responsibilities has been to help run a clinic giving long-acting anti-psychotic 'depot' injections to stabilise patients diagnosed*

*continued overleaf . . .*

continued . . .

> *with schizophrenia so that they can live in the community. Martin, a patient delegated to Franco by his mentor, has a history of psychotic behaviour. If he does not take his medication he has been known to believe he is 'John the Baptist' and walk naked through town to 'cleanse the souls of sinners' or try to 'fly to heaven' and fall from an upstairs window, breaking his arm. Despite agreeing to come to the clinic, Martin repeatedly fails to attend. Franco alerts his mentor and they do a home visit to administer the injection, which involves getting past Martin's sometimes hostile and paranoid mother (who thinks they are poisoning her son). Martin reassures her, saying, 'It's alright Mum. I'll have the injection.' He apologises for not making the clinic, saying he didn't feel like going. Franco offers to go with him to the clinic next time but Martin says he'd rather have the injection at home. They chat about philosophy for a while as both share an interest in it. Franco leaves feeling frustrated, as he thinks Martin would benefit from getting out more and talking to other people, and he is disappointed he has failed to help him do this.*

Franco's mentor asks him to visualise what might have happened if he had not alerted him that Martin had missed his appointment and they had not followed up by seeing him at home. Franco accepts he played his part in ensuring Martin's psychotic symptoms remain controlled. The mentor then praises Franco for his commitment to helping Martin, his ability to talk to him about things the mentor does not know much about, and his resourcefulness in trying to negotiate a new way of getting Martin out of the house to attend the clinic. They also reflect on how seeing the home situation supports theory about dysfunctional 'double-bind' relationships sometimes found between parents and patients prone to schizophrenia (Koopmans, 1997). The mentor points out that while the mother may not seem 'normal', she has never required compulsory treatment and that her suspicions are those of an anxious mother being protective of her son. Acknowledging this and reassuring her that the injection is good for Martin can help to gain her co-operation.

Whichever field of nursing you are studying and practising in, you, like Franco, are likely to face challenges in collaborating with patients and families; having a supportive mentor will be helpful in this respect. Activity 2.7 asks you to reflect on related issues you have come across.

## Activity 2.7                                    *Reflection*

Take a moment to think about any difficulties that you have experienced in collaborating with patients and their families. Describe the circumstances as well as you can and then examine the reasons for it. See if you can think of a new way to consult and negotiate with those concerned to gain their co-operation in achieving previously agreed aims or new revised aims.

*As this is for you to review your own experience, there is no answer included, but please discuss your responses with your mentor.*

Recognising the important contribution that patients and relatives can make, consulting with them to facilitate this and negotiating ways of overcoming problems are endorsed by health policy. The Department of Health's *Expert Patients Programme* (DH, 2006a) is a case in point as patients, particularly with long-term conditions, are seen as 'experts' in understanding and managing their own care needs, and online resources are available to help them do this. Hence, health professionals can both learn from and support patients in collaborative decision-making.

# Collaborating with other health professionals

As in collaborative decision-making with patients, the need for nurses to recognise the important contribution of other health professionals in person/patient-centred care is also emphasised in *The Code: Standards of conduct, performance and ethics for nurses and midwives*:

> *Work with others to protect and promote the health and well-being of those in your care, their families and carers, and the wider community.*

> *Share information with your colleagues.*

> *Work effectively as part of a team.*
> (NMC, 2008, p5)

Collaborative clinical decision-making complements the aim in recent health policy to integrate patient-centred health and social care, hospital services and community services more effectively to raise efficiency and quality, and reduce errors associated with fragmented care (DH, 2006b). It is, therefore, important to understand the roles of other health professionals and refer to them patients who need their expertise. The use of integrated care pathways (ICPs) as structured, evidence-based, multidisciplinary care plans to guide high quality care for specific clinical conditions (Campbell et al., 1998) is an example of how to acknowledge, harness and co-ordinate the contributions of different health professionals. Chapter 5 discusses ICPs in more detail. Without collaborative clinical decision-making, care is not responsive to patients' or the wider public's expressed needs; different health professionals, social care and other agencies work in isolation from one another (even when attending to the same patient); there is a lack of communication, integration and co-ordination of services they provide, necessary referrals are not made and, sadly, sometimes tragically, poor-quality care is likely to result from this. The case study below explores these issues.

## Case study: Tragic outcome of non-collaboration

*In 2007 the bodies of a 38-year-old woman and her 18-year-old daughter were found in the woman's car after she is believed to have set it alight. The woman had borderline learning difficulties and her daughter had severe learning difficulties with an estimated mental age of just 4. They were stigmatised because of the daughter's obvious disability, and they suffered years of sustained hate, abuse, persecution and terror day and night from gangs of local youths. In the year before they died, the mother complained to the police thirteen times but no action was taken either against the offenders or to help the mother when she expressed suicidal intentions if the abuse did not stop.*

*In the aftermath of the tragedy it was concluded that serious failures had occurred in: not prioritising the complaint; treating each complaint separately and not recognising the persistent pattern of abuse; not sharing*

*continued overleaf . . .*

*continued* . . . .

*information between agencies (police, social services, council housing officers); not referring the mother to get medical or nursing help to relieve the burden of caring for her daughter; and not referring her for a mental health assessment when she said she was going to kill herself because she could not cope any more.*

In this case study there was no collaborative decision-making. If there had been, the tragedy could have been prevented. When the mother repeatedly consulted the police, they did not make an adequate risk assessment, no effective strategy was negotiated to address her concerns, and there was no co-operation with health and social care agencies, who were not alerted. It is one of many tragedies in recent years where the most vulnerable people in society have been let down by a lack of responsive, collaborative and integrated care, focused on the person's needs and preferences, by health and social care agencies in hospital or in the community. It is a reminder for nurses, other health and social care professionals, and community agencies that further tragedies will happen if there is no effective safety net of collaborative decision-making. Sometimes, as nurses, we could do more to let other agencies know what different skills and services we can offer patients. For example, other professions have said that they value the contribution of the community learning disability nursing service (Powell and Murray, 2004); if a referral had been made to support the family in the case study, the outcome might have been different.

It is probable that each of the health and social care and community agencies implicated in recent tragedies will have had a mission statement committed to providing a high quality service to all members of the public regardless of age, gender, ethnicity, culture or religion. Very often statistics are used to suggest that these organisations are being effective in the vast number of cases they deal with. Indeed, some people argue that nurses can be more effective in their decision-making if they understand and apply statistics. The main strength of collaborative clinical decision-making in nursing is that it reminds us we are dealing with human beings who have a complex range of continually changing needs, which can only be partially represented or addressed by the rhetoric of mission statements or the science of decision analysis models. In this sense, nursing theory – by focusing on good interpersonal relationships, addressing bio–psycho–social–spiritual needs and offering holistic human caring – remains highly relevant.

# Quality care through collaboration

If we do not collaborate adequately with service users, we cannot: make accurate assessments of their health problems; ensure they are informed and consent to proposed care; know what their needs and preferences are; or know what their experience of the healthcare provided is. If we do not collaborate adequately with the healthcare team or other agencies, we cannot contribute to the delivery of effective, integrated, high quality inter-professional care. Collaborative decision-making by service users and healthcare team members is, therefore, vital for high quality care.

# Integrating collaboration with patients, families and other health professionals

In clinical practice nurses have to collaborate simultaneously with patients, their families, other health professionals and various agencies all the time because complex health problems need a co-ordinated approach. This is illustrated in the following case study.

## Case study: Collaborating with child, parents and healthcare team

*Sanjeev is a seven-year-old boy admitted to a children's ward in great pain and distress, having broken his arm falling from a bouncy castle at his friend's birthday party. Alison, a third-year student, welcomes him and his parents to the ward and asks a couple of other children to come and say hello. Alison asks Sanjeev to tell her what happened and where it hurts, without touching his arm, in order not to exacerbate his pain. She can see that the left forearm is crooked and that there are no bones protruding through the skin, which is consistent with a 'greenstick' fracture. Alison tells Sanjeev he is very brave and clever to use his right arm to support and protect the left one, and that she will ask the doctor to see him so they can mend his arm and stop it hurting.*

*X-rays confirm fractures to the radius and ulna bones in the left arm. Alison applies an anaesthetic skin patch to Sanjeev's right arm so that he won't feel the needle when given an anaesthetic before surgery. The parents try to comfort Sanjeev, but he screams and fights against the injection so the anaesthetist gives gas via a face mask; Sanjeev inhales and loses consciousness so they can proceed with surgery. Alison can see the parents are upset and talks to them. They express remorse for letting him go to the party not realising it had an unsupervised bouncy castle that caused their son such a serious injury. They are also sorry they could not calm Sanjeev down during the anaesthesia when he was so frightened.*

*Alison informs them that these injuries are common, young bones are usually quick to heal, Sanjeev will be given pain relief after surgery, and he can go home in a day or two once they are sure there no after-effects from the anaesthetic or complications with the arm or its protective cast. She shows them the family area where they can sit down and have a cup of tea while they are waiting. She mentions how they felt during the anaesthesia to her mentor who asks her to tell the anaesthetist when surgery is over, which, nervously, she does. The anaesthetist then goes to see the parents to explain that although they try to be as gentle as possible, it is not unusual for a frightened child in a lot of pain to be resistant. But the operation went well, Sanjeev is now alert, his pain is controlled, and they can go and see him.*

In this case study, Alison demonstrated effective collaborative clinical decision-making with patients, families, and other health professionals by consulting with:

- Sanjeev in identifying the nature and cause of his injury;
- the parents in acknowledging and reporting their concerns, and in keeping them informed so they would know how to support their son;
- the inter-professional healthcare team (nurse mentor, orthopaedic doctor, radiographer and anaesthetist) in caring for Sanjeev and diagnosing and treating his broken arm.

In doing so, Alison showed how to link theory and practice in relating caring, holistic and interpersonal values, knowledge and skills to collaborative clinical decision-making.

Sometimes you might be worried that your own role is less clear or possibly threatened by the roles and expertise of other professionals. One way of assessing the relevance of nurses' expertise within inter-professional care is to summarise the key elements of nursing and then cross-reference these with the case study examples of collaborative clinical decision-making. As mentioned in Chapter 1, nurses identified ten conceptions of nursing (as well as perceptions of clinical decision-making) in a research study (Standing, 2005). They are called conceptions rather than concepts as they represent nurses' own growing understanding of their professional identity acquired through experience, as opposed to purely academic, theoretical knowledge.

Table 2.1 sets out the conceptions of nursing that Alison was applying in her care of Sanjeev and how they relate to collaborative decision-making.

| Conceptions of nursing | Collaborative clinical decision-making |
|---|---|
| Caring | Comforting Sanjeev by telling him he is brave and clever. |
| Listening and being there | Enabling Sanjeev to explain how he was injured. Enabling parents to talk about their feelings. |
| Practical procedures | Pre-operative procedures, e.g. anaesthetic gel skin patch. |
| Knowledge and understanding | Pain control, pre-/post-operative care, care of broken arm, developmental psychology, exclude non-accidental injury. |
| Communicating | Talking softly to Sanjeev, introducing him to other children, orientate parents to ward, explain care plan and prognosis. |
| Patience | Remaining calm when Sanjeev is screaming and fighting off attempts to give him an intravenous anaesthetic. |
| Teamwork | Referral to orthopaedic surgeon, arranging X-ray, reporting parents' concerns to mentor and to the anaesthetist. |
| Paperwork and electronic record | Ensuring parents have signed consent form before surgery. |
| Empathising and non-judgemental | Appreciate Sanjeev's distress at his painful injury when he was supposed to be having fun at a party. Understanding the parents' guilt feelings, anger and concerns. |
| Professional | Courteous to parents/colleagues, competent assessment of injury, conscientious and diligent in caring for family. |

*Table 2.1: Integrating collaborative clinical decision-making with conceptions of nursing*

Table 2.1 suggests that key characteristics (conceptions of nursing) identified by nurses (in putting into words the nature of their own professional identity) complement the integrated collaborative decision-making with patient/family and health professionals in the case study. Activity 2.8 invites you to apply the same process to your experience of healthcare teamwork.

---

### Activity 2.8 — *Teamwork*

Identify an example from your own area of practice as a nurse collaborating with patients and relatives plus other health professionals. Use the same format as Table 2.1 to draw up your own table and try to match and integrate your examples of collaborative decision-making with the conceptions of nursing. Reflect on whether it is useful to relate ideas about what nursing is to collaborative decisions nurses make with other healthcare professionals.

*As this is for your own personal reflection there is no specimen answer included, but it might be interesting for you to ask colleagues in practice/other nursing students to work through the same activity and then compare notes on this.*

---

Hopefully, you will have found that Activity 2.8 has helped to reinforce the importance of good teamwork for effective, collaborative decision-making with patients, families and other health professionals. You may also have found that cross-referencing conceptions of nursing helps you to illustrate and validate your own developing professional identity while working together with others. The conceptions of nursing are also cross-referenced to different decision-making skills in each of the remaining chapters.

---

### Chapter summary

Of all the different perceptions of significant clinical decision-making identified by nurses, collaborative decision-making received the most support (Standing, 2005). It therefore seemed the logical place to begin our exploration of nurses' clinical decision-making in this book. This chapter argued that collaborative clinical decision-making involves consultation, negotiation and co-operation with patients, relatives, inter-professional colleagues and other agencies. Its main strengths are in promoting responsive, relevant, high quality and integrated patient/person-centred care through a good nurse–patient relationship and effective teamwork. Weaknesses include collusion, a negative type of collaboration; for example, by not helping vulnerable people we are colluding with those who abuse them. We discussed how to apply collaborative clinical decision-making, first with patients and their families, then with other health professionals, and finally, how to combine them in providing high quality, integrated inter-professional healthcare. In doing so, the nature of our own professional identity as nurses was outlined, and this was shown to be well suited and equipped for collaborative clinical decision-making.

## Activities: brief outline answers

### Activity 2.1 Decision-making (page 21)

You may have identified the following aspects of collaborative decision-making.

- Joint decision between two or more people.
- Identification of a shared aim.
- Working together to achieve the aim.
- Consultation, negotiation and co-operation.

### Activity 2.2 Reflection (page 21)

You may have reflected on the following aspects of collusion.

- Secretive alliance promoting alternative agenda.
- Inconsistency between stated beliefs and actions.
- Actions undermining prevailing social or moral values.
- Lack of confidence to challenge inappropriate behaviour.

### Activity 2.4 Critical thinking (page 24)

As mentioned earlier, critical thinking involves applying logical reasoning, evaluating relevant evidence, and being aware of gaps in knowledge regarding beliefs, intentions and actions.

You may have thought of the following (linking collaboration and evidence-based practice).

- Eliciting patients' signs, symptoms and preferences is a source of evidence.
- Giving rationale for care helps patients make informed decisions about consent.
- Patient feedback can help to determine whether treatment is being effective.
- Healthcare team supplies evidence to support diagnosis, e.g. X-ray of broken bone.
- Healthcare team members share experience and research knowledge about treatment options.
- Family and friends can provide helpful information about patients' health.

### Activity 2.5 Communication (page 25)

You may have identified the following aspects of consulting with patients:

- Focusing attention on patients rather than on your own need for a chat.
- Eliciting views and preferences regarding patients' health needs.
- Engaging patients in collaborative, clinical decision-making.
- Informing patient-centred care that is relevant to their needs.
- Explaining treatment options, enabling patients' informed consent.
- Answering patients' questions and giving health promotion advice.

### Activity 2.6 Leadership and management (page 27)

You may have referred to the following obstacles to collaborative decision-making.

- Pressurised clinical environment encourages task-orientated care.
- Standardised procedures may be used to support a medical model of care.
- Fatigue may result in nurses lacking energy to talk with patients.
- Talking to patients might be seen as shirking other responsibilities.
- Nurses may not feel confident in communicating with patients.
- Collaborative decision-making is not customary practice in that area.

## Further reading

**Goodman, B and Clemow, R** (2010) *Nursing and Collaborative Practice* (2nd edn). Exeter: Learning Matters.

A very useful introduction to collaborating with others in nursing, including: relevant policy developments, service-user participation and inter-professional teamwork.

**Reed, A** (2011) *Patient and Carer Participation in Nursing.* Exeter: Learning Matters.

Clear guidance on maximising the quality of patients' experience through person-centred partnership.

## Useful websites

**www.expertpatients.co.uk**

A site mainly for patients to access resources to help with problem solving and decision-making in managing their own care (also useful for health professionals).

# Chapter 3
# Using observation
# to inform decisions

```
                                                   NMC Standards for Pre-registration Nursing Education
```

This chapter will address the following competencies:

**Domain 2: Communication and interpersonal skills**

4. All nurses must recognise when people are anxious or in distress and respond effectively, using therapeutic principles, to promote their well-being, manage personal safety
   and resolve conflict. They must use effective communication strategies and negotiation
   techniques to achieve best outcomes, respecting the dignity and human rights of all
   concerned. They must know when to consult a third party and how to make referrals
   for advocacy, mediation or arbitration.

**Domain 3: Nursing practice and decision-making**

7. All nurses must be able to recognise and interpret signs of normal and deteriorating
   mental and physical health and respond promptly to maintain or improve the health
   and comfort of the service user, acting to keep them and others safe.

```
                                                                   NMC Essential Skills Clusters
```

This chapter will address the following ESCs:

**Cluster: Care, compassion and communication**

6. People can trust the newly registered graduate nurse to engage therapeutically and
   actively listen to their needs and concerns, responding using skills that are helpful,
   providing information that is clear, accurate, meaningful and free from jargon.
   *By the first progression point:*
   ii. Records information accurately and clearly on the basis of observation and
       communication.

**Cluster: Organisational aspects of care**

9. People can trust the newly registered graduate nurse to treat them as partners and work
   with them to make a holistic and systematic assessment of their needs; to develop a personalised plan that is based on mutual understanding and respect for their individual
   situation promoting health and well-being, minimising risk of harm and promoting
   their safety at all times.

*continued opposite . . .*

*continued . . .*

*By the second progression point:*

vi.  Measures and documents vital signs under supervision and responds appropriately to findings outside the normal range.

*By entry to the register:*

xxi. Measures, documents and interprets vital signs and acts autonomously and appropriately on findings.

10. People can trust the newly registered graduate nurse to deliver nursing interventions and evaluate their effectiveness against the agreed assessment and care plan.

    *By the second progression point:*

    v.  Detects, records, reports and responds appropriately to signs of deterioration or improvement.

11. People can trust the newly registered graduate nurse to safeguard children and adults from vulnerable situations and support and protect them from harm.

    *By entry to the register:*

    v.  Recognises and responds when people are in vulnerable situations and at risk, or in need of support and protection.

17. People can trust the newly registered graduate nurse to work safely under pressure and maintain the safety of service users at all times.

    *By the first progression point:*

    i.  Recognises when situations are becoming unsafe and reports appropriately.

19. People can trust the newly registered nurse to work to prevent and resolve conflict and maintain a safe environment.

    *By the first progression point:*

    i.  Recognises signs of aggression and responds appropriately to keep self and others safe.

## Chapter aims

By the end of this chapter, you should be able to:

* explain how observations inform clinical decision-making;
* give examples of decisions informed by patient observation;
* apply observation to detect physical and psychological signs;
* relate observation to patient assessment and evaluating care.
* use observation in recognising and responding to health risks.
* appreciate the importance of observation in decision-making.

# Introduction

Without observation, patient-centred clinical judgement and decision-making in evidence-based nursing care is not possible. It is therefore vital for nurses to apply effective observational skills.

---

### Case study: Destined to be a nurse

*When asked to reflect on reasons why she had chosen to study nursing, Serena described an early childhood memory where she had recognised that another child needed medical attention:*

*'When I was seven I was playing outside my home and I saw a neighbour's child fall down as he was running across the road. He had sliced open the skin underneath his chin, which had hit the kerb as he fell, and it was bleeding. The boy looked unsteady when he got up and he was crying. There were grown-ups who saw what happened and lots of other children around but everyone seemed to be in a panic. I just grabbed the kid, held him under the chin and walked with him to see his mother. So people said, "She's a nurse" and it's just stuck from that moment.'*

---

Serena's childhood memory nicely illustrates the importance of **observation in clinical decision-making**, and how an ability to link the two is associated with being a nurse by members of the public. Observation is important because without it you cannot see if anything is wrong with a person. However, it is limited unless followed by appropriate judgement, decision-making and action to address the problem by relieving pain or suffering, and promoting healing and recovery. For example, the 'grown-ups' saw what had happened to the boy but did not take any action. Perhaps they did not think the injury was as serious as Serena thought, and if she had not intervened, the boy would possibly have made his own way home to be cared for by his mother. Knowing whether to act on observations in healthcare is therefore very much a 'judgement call'.

Young Serena showed how observation can be effectively used to inform decision-making by:

- being alert to changing situations and any associated health risks;
- recognising the boy was distressed and nobody was helping him;
- remaining calm in responding and attending to the boy after the accident;
- assessing the boy's physical injury and his emotional reaction;
- applying first-aid to minimise blood loss by supporting his chin;
- transferring the boy to his mother for further treatment and comfort;
- reporting observations and reasons for decisions and actions;
- exercising leadership, inspiring others to have confidence in her.

This chapter explores nurses' use of observation to inform decisions, starting by clarifying what this entails and its relevance to evidence-based nursing. Observation of patients' physical and mental health is described, and examples of assessment and evaluating care are given. The pros and cons of manual versus automated observations of patients' vital signs, and their potential use as an 'early warning' system to predict and prevent deteriorating health, are also outlined. The importance of accurately recording observations is then emphasised. Finally, the strengths and weaknesses of using observation to inform decisions are summarised.

# What does using observation to inform decisions mean?

Observation is usually associated with using our eyes in noticing what is happening around us, just as Serena did when she saw the boy fall. We also use other senses to get information about situations we find ourselves in; for example, if Serena had not seen the boy fall, she would still have known something was wrong because she could hear him crying. Blind or partially sighted people rely more on hearing, feeling their way around using a white stick, or being accompanied by a guide dog or someone else to see for them. Conversely, the deaf or partially deaf compensate by relying more on sight in 'lip reading' and using sign language. Those of us fortunate to have good eyesight and hearing can learn from those with sensory impairment by making fuller use of the senses we possess. For example, we can emulate deaf people by paying closer attention to 'body language' when interacting with others, just as Serena did when recognising the boy was distressed and others 'seemed to be in a panic'. We also use the senses of smell and taste every day – when we are judging whether our food or drink is safe to consume, for example. Hence, observation is not restricted to what we can see – it involves the use of all the senses in processing stimuli. In Activity 3.1 you are asked to note the different sensory stimuli that you are currently experiencing.

---

## Activity 3.1         *Reflection*

Take a few moments to identify different stimuli you might be sensing while reading this chapter.

### Sight
* What do you think of the design and layout of the book?
* Are the printed words too small, the right size, or too big?
* Do you need to wear spectacles or contact lenses to read?
* Are you recalling any images from previous experiences?
* What things catch your eye and distract you from reading?

### Hearing
* Do the pages sound crisp or floppy when you turn them?
* Are you reading out loud or silently to yourself?
* If reading silently, can you 'hear' your own internal voice?
* Is it possible for you to read while listening to music?
* Do you find other noises can distract you from reading?
* What background sounds can you hear at the moment?
* Can you hear yourself breathing?

*continued overleaf . . .*

---

*continued . . .*

## Touch

- Does the book feel pleasant or unpleasant to hold?
- Have you ever suffered a paper cut when turning a page?
- Are you happy to use library books read by many others?
- If it is your own book, would you let others read it or not?
- Do you need to walk about to relieve pressure areas?

## Smell

- Do the pages smell new and fresh or old and musty?
- Does the atmosphere seem pleasant or a bit stale?
- What aromas are you able to detect at this time?
- Is there a smell of cooking wafting from a kitchen?

## Taste

- Do you like to eat or drink while you are reading?
- What, if anything, can you taste at the moment?

*As this activity is intended to help you to identify different sensory stimuli you are personally experiencing, only you can know what the answers are, so no outline answer is provided.*

By completing Activity 3.1, you should be able to appreciate that at any one time our senses are being continually bombarded by a wide range of stimuli, even if we are sitting quietly trying to read. Much of this goes unnoticed since many sensory stimuli are filtered out of consciousness as they are deemed irrelevant to the task at hand. This can be helpful and unhelpful in relation to decision-making. For example, your decision to try to learn something useful by reading this chapter is helped if you are able to ignore distractions such as a neighbour playing heavy metal music at full volume. On the other hand, being unaware of how to control distractions when finding a place you find conducive to learning is unhelpful, as you are less likely to be successful at completing the tasks you set yourself. Observation skills are useful for knowing how to focus attention on important things and for recognising, and avoiding where possible, unhelpful stimuli that are an unnecessary distraction. Sometimes it is important to be distracted from what you are doing – it is clearly unwise to carry on reading if you smell burning, see smoke and hear the fire alarm. What is considered to be a priority can, therefore, suddenly change. As nurses caring for patients, we need to be even more vigilant in developing and applying the observation skills needed to accurately inform decisions that promote health and minimise risks.

# Relevance of observation in evidence-based nursing

For the purposes of this chapter observation means:

*using all the senses (sight, hearing, touch, smell, taste) to assess patients' bio–psycho–social–spiritual well being, check if they need assistance, monitor their vital signs, review results of investigations, record response to treatment and report concerns.*

As we saw in Chapter 1, observation skills have always been associated with nursing. For example, Florence Nightingale used them in developing and applying evidence for the benefits of good hygiene and sanitation in her environmental health theory. A recent trend has been to promote evidence-based practice while regarding nursing perceptions as less reliable evidence. The intention behind this policy is to promote high quality care that is based upon sound research evidence as opposed to local custom and practice that fails to keep up with new developments. However, the assumption that what nurses do in everyday practice cannot be trusted results in 'throwing the baby out with the bathwater' if our observations are no longer considered valid. It is good to update knowledge ('throw bathwater') but not good to deskill nurses or undermine professional identity ('throw baby') developed by *observing* and interacting with patients. This chapter argues that observation is an important part of well-informed evidence-based nursing.

Nurses' professional code and standards of conduct states, *You must deliver care based on the best available evidence or best practice* (NMC, 2008, p7). The idea that some forms of evidence might be considered better than others (in terms of being more rigorously researched or tested) has led to the development of hierarchies of evidence such as the one shown in Table 3.1. This assumes that level 1 is the strongest and level 6 is the weakest type of evidence in the range.

A quick look at Table 3.1 indicates that nursing observations do not feature as a specific form of evidence in the hierarchy although, arguably, level 6 is informed by practitioners' observations. Observation is vital in carrying out research referred to in levels 1–4; otherwise there would be no results to report, and no research-based NICE (National Institute of Health and Clinical

| Level | Description |
|-------|-------------|
| 1 | Systematic reviews of randomised controlled trials |
| 2 | Randomised controlled trials |
| 3 | Non-randomised experiments |
| 4 | Non-experimental research |
| 5 | Expert opinion and NICE guidelines |
| 6 | Views of peers/inter-professional colleagues |

*Table 3.1: Evidence-based nursing practice: hierarchy of evidence*

Source: Adapted from 'The hierarchy of evidence', available on the Evidence Based Nursing Practice website www.ebnp.co.uk/The%20Hierarchy%20of%20Evidence.htm

Excellence) clinical guidelines published (level 5). However, research observations differ from nursing observations: the main focus is to generate knowledge rather than deliver care; they are constrained by the specific research questions being asked; and it is often recommended that the results can be applied to other areas that were not observed or included in the research study. The hierarchy prompts nurses to value research observations from elsewhere as more reliable types of evidence than their own observations of patient care.

This can place nurses in a bit of a quandary as we are required to be observant, attentive and responsive in giving relevant 'person-centred care' (NMC, 2010a) while, wherever possible, applying rigorous research evidence that has not directly involved the patients we are caring for. Being both patient-centred and evidence-based can seem like trying to 'fit a square peg into a round hole' if nursing observations are not considered a valid form of evidence, or if in applying research findings, patients' individual needs and preferences are not addressed. Activity 3.2 asks you to think about how observation skills contributed to Serena's decision-making in the case study and whether her actions are supported by more authoritative sources of evidence.

---

### Activity 3.2                                           *Decision-making*

*Hint: Remember that decision-making involves choosing a course of action from the available options, an ability to explain the reasoning behind it, and being accountable for the outcome.*

Look back at the description of the case study where Serena helped the boy who had hurt himself and try to answer the following questions.

1. How did Serena know that anything was wrong?
2. What were the different options available to Serena?
3. Why do you think she chose to intervene as described?
4. How might Serena's actions have affected the boy's recovery?
5. What theory or research might support Serena's decision-making?

*There are some possible answers at the end of the chapter.*

---

Now that you have completed Activity 3.2, we should be 'on the same page' in that you can see that observations we make about people in our care are vital sources of evidence. If we do not act on these observations, patients can suffer harm, which could sometimes be fatal. It may seem a bit odd that the carer in the case study is so young, and you might, understandably, feel reluctant to compare your skills and experience with those of a seven-year-old. However, it makes the point that someone with no professional education in healthcare is able to recognise the need to respond to an emergency, and do so in an appropriate manner (even if they are unable to understand or explain all of the principles they are applying). This reinforces the importance of our own observations as nurses in caring for people and how they contribute to our professional knowledge and skills, in addition to formal education, theory and research.

As students you might also expect (as Serena did) that more experienced people – for example, your clinical mentor – will know what to do and guide you in facing challenging situations.

Decision-making requires more than knowing what to do in a given situation, of course – you also need to know why you are taking a particular action, and be able to explain and justify it. This is where we need to link theory and practice by relating our nursing observations and experience to theoretical principles and more scientific forms of evidence. Your mentors and role models will demonstrate how to do this, and as you progress through your programme you will find it easier to integrate theory and practice in this respect. In doing so you will discover a way to resolve the quandary of being attentive and responsive in giving localised patient-centred care, and at the same time ensuring that up-to-date relevant national and international research evidence is applied to practice.

In summary, we can 'change the bathwater without losing the baby' and find a way of making 'square pegs and round holes' more compatible, by acknowledging the following points.

- Nursing observations are valid forms of evidence to inform decision-making because they are patient-centred and enable us to quickly assess and respond to health risks.
- Research evidence is rigorously developed and tested accumulated knowledge that goes beyond that found via personal or local experience, to inform healthcare decisions.
- Nursing observations can be enhanced by applying research evidence in relation to the different assessment/decision-making tools or clinical treatment guidelines we can use.
- Research evidence will remain 'on a library shelf' unless nursing observations are used to identify its relevance to inform and support our decision-making in patient-centred care.

There is now a growing understanding that various forms of evidence have to be acknowledged because different types of problems or circumstances call for different types of knowledge and skills to be applied (Rycroft-Malone et al., 2004). This challenges the concept of a hierarchy as each type of evidence has its own strengths and applications; for example, non-experimental methods such as qualitative research offer more in-depth understanding of people's experience than randomised controlled trials. In addition to the evidence shown in Table 3.1, Ellis (2010) identifies practice knowledge, experience and patient preference as important influences in nursing decisions, all of which incorporate nurses observing, listening to and interacting with patients. In relating the principles of evidence-based practice to systematic **problem solving** in patient-centred nursing care, Hek and Moule (2006) describe five key stages. These are summarised below with a nursing example to demonstrate how they might be applied.

1. Identify a nursing problem and make it into a specific question (*e.g. patient prescribed large tablets cannot swallow them – is there an alternative way to give the medicine?*).
2. Search literature/other sources to find answer to your question (*talk to mentor who advises you to check whether the British National Formulary (BNF) has information on this*).
3. Critically evaluate rigour and relevance of the evidence you find (*find up-to-date edition of BNF, which indicates the medicine can also be given in syrup form*).
4. Select, apply best evidence to address patient need/preference (*tell doctor of problem and possible solution, doctor agrees to prescribe syrup so patient can take medicine*).
5. Evaluate patient outcome after the evidence-based intervention (*patient is able to swallow the syrup and is happy that an alternative to the tablets has been found*).

Systematic problem solving and decision-making in nursing is discussed in more detail in Chapter 4. In the meantime, to help you self-assess how much sense you make of what has been discussed so far, Activity 3.3 asks you to think about how nursing observations might contribute to evidence-based practice using the five stages referred to by Hek and Moule.

---

**Activity 3.3**                    *Evidence-based practice and research*

*Hint: Assess what each stage does plus their collective contribution to patient-centred care.*

Look at Hek and Moule's five stages of evidence-based practice and answer these questions.

1. Which stages are more strongly associated with nursing observations and why?
2. What do you need to do to access evidence that helps tackle nursing problems?
3. How is research or other evidence nurses find related to patient-centred care?

*There are some possible answers at the end of the chapter.*

---

For the purposes of this book, evidence-based practice means never being satisfied you 'know it all' and making sure you use critical thinking skills to continually search, access, critique, apply and evaluate the most relevant up-to-date sources/types of information to guide clinical judgement/decision-making in giving the highest-quality patient-centred care we can. In discussing the relevance of observation to evidence-based nursing, it was argued that nurses' observations are valid forms of evidence in their own right and that they enable us to identify, apply and evaluate other evidence, including research, in patient-centred care. Nursing observations are a window into the world of the patients we care for and interact with, using all of our senses. Research evidence is a window into the wider world of accumulated current knowledge that we tap into to develop our knowledge and understanding, and to enhance the quality of care we give patients. Other types of evidence also inform our practice, including feedback from patients, peers, mentors and inter-professional colleagues, informative text-books, and relevant clinical guidelines. Evidence is, therefore, any kind of information that is used to support reasoning, problem solving, clinical judgement and decision-making, including *observations*, feedback, policy, theory and research.

# Observations used to monitor physical health

As human beings the capacity to sustain life is dependent on our ability to address biological needs, including breathing, maintaining blood flow to all our major organs, eating and drinking, eliminating waste, protecting ourselves from injury or disease, exercising and resting. All these activities can be monitored through nursing observations of patients in our care, enabling us to decide whether any intervention is necessary to help them maintain their vital functions. In order to make accurate observations we need to learn the correct techniques and how to use relevant equipment. To appreciate the significance of the observations, we need a good understanding of relevant anatomy and physiology, and how to distinguish normal from abnormal functioning. We then have to decide whether our observations require further action, which might include double-checking results, increasing the frequency of observations, reporting changes to the clinical manager, helping a patient with heat stroke to cool down, elevating the bottom of the bed to help return blood to the heart for a patient with low blood pressure, or calling for emergency help if a patient stops breathing. It is vital our observations are not considered ritualistic, routine tasks or 'ends in themselves' but as valuable sources of information to assess patients' health and guide decision-making. This is illustrated in the case study below.

## Case study: Reporting alarming change in vital signs

*Lucy is a second-year student nurse on an orthopaedic ward who is asked to observe and record the vital signs of the patients she is helping to care for. Miranda, aged 25, was knocked off her motorcycle by a van whose driver did not see her, and she has a hairline fracture on the back of her skull, a fractured pelvis, and a compound fracture of the tibia and fibula in her left leg. Medical assessment of Miranda indicates her skull and pelvis should heal by themselves but that nurses need to closely observe her for signs of neurological damage (e.g. eyes/pupils not reacting to light, loss of consciousness) or internal bleeding (e.g. low blood pressure, increased respiration and heart rate). Miranda's leg fractures were realigned by screwing pins into her tibia/shinbone that protrude eight centimetres from her skin and support two metal 'external fixators' (a bit like scaffolding). Before Miranda left the operating theatre, a sterile dressing and bandage was applied to the wound (caused by fractured bones breaking through her skin during the accident).*

*It is now three days since surgery and so far Miranda has been progressing reasonably well. She is nursed in bed with her left leg elevated to reduce swelling and she has regular painkillers. Miranda's temperature has been above average (37.7–38.4 degrees centigrade). Lucy's mentor says it might be the body working overtime to heal after trauma but it needs careful monitoring. Other vital signs are within the normal range. The next time Lucy checks Miranda's temperature she is shocked to find it is 40.8 degrees. She wonders if it is a faulty reading, although it is the same device as before (infrared digital aural thermometer) that she placed in Miranda's left ear as she usually does. Lucy tries again in the right ear, and gets the same result. She asks Miranda how she feels; she replies that she feels cold and she appears to be shivering. Lucy gets a blanket for her and brings a different infrared digital aural thermometer to double-check if the previous device was faulty. This time the reading is 41 degrees centigrade so Lucy records it on Miranda's observation chart together with her pulse and respiration rate, which show a slight increase, and her blood pressure, which remains stable. Lucy tells her mentor about the change in Miranda's condition. The mentor confirms Miranda's temperature is 41 degrees and alerts the medical team. They decide that there is a risk Miranda's leg is infected and that it could spread to the bloodstream (septicaemia). There is also a possibility the leg may have to be amputated if the infection does not respond to treatment. They take Miranda back to theatre to thoroughly clean her leg and change the dressing in sterile conditions, and they start her on a course of intravenous antibiotics. The antibiotics are effective and the infection subsides. Miranda's leg wound heals, tibia and fibula mend following more orthopaedic and plastic surgery, and six months late, she can walk unassisted again.*

The case study shows how valuable nursing observations are in early detection and treatment of potentially serious health risks to patients. Lucy did not simply check and record temperature unthinkingly; she was constantly reviewing the significance of observations she made regarding Miranda's health status, and acting upon them if they appeared unusual, as follows.

- Checking with her mentor when the earlier temperature is over one degree above average.
- Repeating digital aural thermometer readings in the other ear to check the result.
- Checking with Miranda how she felt and giving her a blanket when shivering.
- Checking the accuracy of the first device by using a second digital aural thermometer.
- Realising that this is a worrying development that she needs to both record and report.
- Checking with her mentor, who confirms the current temperature is four degrees above average.
- Prompting her mentor to inform the medical team, who treat the infection, which helps the leg to heal.

This demonstrates good practice in carrying out regular observations of patients' vital signs to recognise and respond to the continually changing health status of those with acute illnesses (NICE, 2007b). If Lucy had not reported Miranda's very high temperature straightaway, the outcome might not have been so positive, as the required medical treatment would have been delayed. It emphasises the importance of nurses being vigilant in carrying out and reporting observations. They are vital in so-called 'track and trigger' or 'early warning' systems where referral to medical care is prompted when specified thresholds are reached (e.g. abnormally high temperature). Using observations to prevent deterioration in this way is strongly endorsed by the National Patient Safety Agency (NPSA, 2007). The NPSA represents the interests of service users and is concerned about instances where patients' health deteriorates without being noticed. The NPSA is also concerned that while automated devices to monitor vital signs are faster, they give less opportunity to observe and interact with patients. It argues that manual, mercury sphygmo-manometers (seldom used now) are more accurate for detecting low blood pressure. Mercury is a poison and such devices are health risks if broken so care is needed if used. When using automated devices to monitor vital signs, the NPSA appeals to nurses to still take time to observe and interact with patients, as Lucy did in checking out how Miranda was feeling.

## Activity 3.4 *Evidence-based practice and research*

Look at the following list of nursing observations and think of all the health risks that each one can help us identify; then use the web/library to search for more evidence and jot down findings for future reference. Discuss with your mentor any procedures you need more practice in.

| Observations | Identifying potential health risks |
|---|---|
| Temperature | |
| Pulse | |
| Respiration | |
| Blood pressure | |
| Oxygen saturation | |
| Urine analysis | |
| Weight | |
| Skin appearance | |

*continued opposite . . .*

*continued . . .*

| Observations | Identifying potential health risks |
|---|---|
| Neurological | |
| Pain chart | |
| Fluid balance | |
| Bowel movement | |

*As this activity is intended to be a self-directed learning experience there is no answer provided but you might also find it useful to talk to your colleagues and compare each other's findings.*

Having looked at physical observations, we turn to those of a more elusive psychological nature.

# Observations to monitor mental health

In many ways observations of mental health are less clear-cut or quantifiable than those used to monitor physical health. However, some of the observations we make of patients' physical health may be relevant when assessing mental health, as the following examples illustrate.

- Anxiety can cause the heart to beat faster than normal (tachycardia) and the person may become aware of an unusual heart rhythm (palpitations) that increases anxiety.
- Anxiety may also cause a person to breathe rapidly and shallowly (hyperventilation).
- Low body weight is sometimes due to a psychological illness called anorexia nervosa or self-neglect associated with depression, psychosis, alcohol or drug addiction.
- Neurological functions (e.g. consciousness, perception, co-ordination) can be disrupted by psychotic delusions or hallucinations, intoxication, or the side-effects of prescribed drugs.

More specific mental health observations focus upon a person's mood, thoughts and behaviour.

## Mood

We all experience a range of emotions – happy, sad, anxious, fearful or angry – but if we get stuck in one, we can become manic, depressed, obsessive, phobic, psychopathic, or a combination of these, such as bi-polar (manic depression) illness with extreme mood swings.

## Thoughts

Who? Where? When? These are the questions with which to start, to see how well orientated and alert a person is. Do they know who they are, where they are, and when they are here (day/month/year)? Simply asking someone what they are thinking can sometimes help them to reveal things about themselves they would not usually volunteer. It is important that we discover if a person has a good grasp of reality or if they have any irrational beliefs such as paranoid delusions that resist any concrete evidence to the contrary. We also need to know how a person's thoughts relate to their moods; for example, what do they think about when they are feeling down and depressed?

# Behaviour

A person's behaviour is something we can observe more directly than their mood or thoughts. It can include how well they communicate with people, relationships with family, friends or others, work or leisure activity, sleep patterns, and how well they look after their personal care. In assessing health risks we need to check if depressive feelings or paranoid thoughts were acted upon in the past, as this makes it more likely the person may harm themselves or others again.

In the following case study, a third-year mental health nurse is on a community placement that includes monitoring the well-being of residents in a hostel following their discharge from hospital.

## Case study: From self-neglect and social isolation to self-care and social interaction

*Phillip (aged 53) has had several admissions to mental health units to be treated for depression and suicidal thoughts. He has always been very shy, and his self-confidence took a further dive when he was made redundant from a computer programming job five years ago. His wife then left him for another man. They have one grown-up son, a sailor on a submarine, who Phillip rarely sees. Phillip now has a part-time job as a maintenance technician at an internet café near the hostel where he lives.*

*Jim, a third-year mental health student, visits Phillip once a week with his mentor to monitor his progress. Jim notices that Phillip's trousers look too big and discovers he has not been eating well since leaving hospital. With his mentor's agreement, Jim asks Phillip if he would like to work with him over the next eight weeks to look at ways of improving his diet.*

*Phillip uses his computer skills to become an expert in counting calories, nutritional properties of different foods, maximum daily levels of salt, sugar and fat to consume, and how to calculate and categorise his body mass index to see if he is underweight, normal or overweight. He keeps in touch with Jim via email and they plan his daily menu a week in advance. Jim goes shopping with Phillip to a local general store on a couple of occasions, and Phillip finds they are quite friendly to him, and goes on his own from that point on. Jim and Phillip also experiment in the communal kitchen with tuna pasta bake, spaghetti bolognaise and chicken curry and rice. This enables Phillip to get to know the other residents better, and they begin to regard him as their 'resident boffin', answering questions about what they are eating and drinking. In exchange, they start to invite Phillip to join them if there is a good film worth watching. At the end of Jim's placement Phillip is eating better, has regained some weight, and feels more self-confident, at ease with other residents.*

As mentioned earlier, physical observations often reveal aspects of a person's mental health. Jim's observation that Phillip's trousers were 'falling off' revealed that he had been neglecting his diet. This gave them both something tangible to work towards and achieve. In doing this, Phillip used his computer expertise to learn new knowledge and skills. These led to making social contact with other residents and local shopkeepers, which increased his self-confidence. This form of therapy focuses on behaviour rather than exploring painful feelings and memories that Phillip evidently had, but which you cannot really do anything about. Jim was relieved he found something he could help Phillip with because he did not know what to say that might help him get over the painful life events he had experienced. The rationale for such activity-based therapy is that actually doing things helps to change your mood and mindset (NICE, 2009).

A key risk factor regarding Phillip's aftercare following discharge from hospital was a possibility he might get so depressed that he could act on the suicidal intentions he had previously expressed. Jim's mentor struck a balance between enabling him to develop his confidence and skills in working with Phillip 'one-to-one', while independently observing and assessing Phillip's progress to ensure any potential suicidal risk was as controlled as it could be. He also talked to Jim about plans he had made with Phillip, the effects of implementing these, and need to record everything he did, including extracts of his email exchanges, as required by the NMC (2008, p8):

*Keep clear and accurate records*
- *You must keep clear and accurate records of the discussions you have, the assessments you make, the treatment and medicines you give and how effective these have been.*
- *You must complete records as soon as possible after an event has occurred.*

Activity 3.5 asks you to critique Jim's involvement in Phillip's mental health care.

---

## Activity 3.5         *Critical thinking*

When discussing ways to assess or monitor a person's mental health, observations of physical signs, mood, thoughts and behaviour were identified. Using these criteria, how would you assess the progress Phillip seemed to make in the eight weeks that Jim was working with him?

*Some possible answers can be found at the end of the chapter.*

---

Table 3.2 relates the case study to observation in decision-making and conceptions of nursing.

| Conceptions of nursing | Observation in clinical decision-making |
|---|---|
| Caring | Jim was concerned Phillip was not looking after himself. |
| Listening and being there | Jim observed Phillip was good with computers and encouraged him to share knowledge he had gained. |
| Practical procedures | Jim helped Phillip to organise menus, plan and execute shopping trips, and prepare various home-cooked meals. |

*continued overleaf . . .*

*Table 3.2: Integrating observation in clinical decision-making and conceptions of nursing*

| Conceptions of nursing | Observation in clinical decision-making |
|---|---|
| Knowledge and understanding | Jim knew his limitations so did not offer Phillip counselling, but focused instead on applying an understanding of nutrition. |
| Communicating | Questioning Phillip about his ill-fitting trousers, agreeing plans to work together to address his dietary problems. |
| Patience | Committed to eight weeks of helping Phillip; understood that progress had to be at a pace he was comfortable with. |
| Teamwork | Worked closely with mentor to oversee the care given. |
| Paperwork and electronic record | Recorded plan of care and progress in achieving goals in case notes, including an audit trail of emails with Phillip. |
| Empathising and non-judgemental | Understood Phillip had lost job and wife, rarely saw son and found relationships difficult, and did not blame him. |
| Professional | Realised that, despite respecting and liking Phillip, he was not his friend. He was a person it was his duty to help. |

*Table 3.2: Continued*

## Chapter summary

This chapter argued that nursing observations are important and valid sources of evidence to inform patient-centred clinical judgement, decision-making and care delivery. It was accepted that such observations may not be as rigorously tested as some forms of research evidence. The key strength of nursing observations are that they focus on what is happening physically and psychologically to the patient, enabling their needs or preferences to be assessed, and the effects of treatment and care evaluated in relation to patient outcomes and satisfaction levels. They have potential in a preventative way to detect early warning signs and respond appropriately to avoid deterioration in patients' health. Nursing observations are also needed to identify questions about addressing patients' needs or improving the quality of care they receive by identifying, accessing, reviewing, applying relevant research results and evaluating their effects. Without nursing observations and related questions, much useful research will remain unused on the 'library shelf'. The weaknesses of nursing observations are that they are subject to individual variations in the skills of the observers and the equipment they use, and that they are by nature localised, and their importance is therefore easily overlooked in the wake of more scientific, quantifiable forms of evidence. Hence it is necessary to apply observations systematically (as discussed in Chapter 4).

## Activities: brief outline answers

### Activity 3.2 Decision-making (page 42)

1. Serena saw the boy fall down, noticed that he was unsteady when he got up, that he had a significant cut underneath his chin, which was bleeding, and that he was crying.
2. Serena could have: carried on with what she was doing as she was not obliged to look after the boy; left it to the grown-ups to decide what to do; let the boy make his own way home to get help; or taken the initiative to help him herself.
3. Serena probably chose to intervene because: she recognised the boy was hurt; nobody else was helping him; he appeared to need medical attention and comforting; she knew where he lived; and she understood his mother was responsible for her son's care.
4. Serena's actions might have helped the boy to begin to recover from the injury by: supporting him under the chin in order to stem blood loss, prevent the wound from gaping, make it easier to suture (if required) and minimise potential scarring; removing him from the roadside where, in his unsteady state, he might be at risk of further injury; and reporting the accident so his mother could arrange medical assessment/treatment if necessary.
5. Serena's decision-making was consistent with the principles of first-aid in: keeping calm when assessing risks; not causing any further harm; removing the boy from danger; giving early intervention; controlling blood loss; comforting the victim who might be dazed or in shock, and transferring him to an appropriate agency for continued care (St John Ambulance et al., 2009).

### Activity 3.3 Evidence-based practice and research (page 44)

1. Stages 1 and 5 because they require nurses to observe patients – in order to identify problems – and to evaluate the effects of research-based interventions, respectively.
2. Identify a problem and make it into a specific question you can search for an answer to.
3. Research evidence is related to patient centred care by: searching for evidence relevant to nursing problems; selecting evidence that helps address patients' needs/preferences; and evaluating patient outcomes regarding the effects of applying the research evidence.

### Activity 3.5 Critical thinking (page 49)

Progress: physical: improved diet, put on weight, clothes fitting better.

Progress: mood: feeling more self-confident and valued by others.

Progress: thoughts: acquired new understanding and expertise regarding nutrition.

Progress: behaviour: able to plan menu, go shopping, cook meals and interact more with others.

## Further reading

**Sharples, K** (2009) *Learning to Learn in Nursing Practice*. Exeter: Learning Matters.

Valuable book that demonstrates how observations of nursing practice offer a rich repertoire to inform learning.

## Useful websites

**www.npsa.nhs.uk**

National Patient Safety Agency (NPSA) website promoting high standards of health and safety in patient care, including effective observation to help prevent deterioration.

# Chapter 4
# Systematic clinical decision-making

*continued opposite . . .*

*continued . . . .*

x.  With the person and under supervision, plans safe and effective care by recording and sharing information based on the assessment.

*By entry to the register:*

xii.  In partnership with the person, their carers and families, makes a holistic, person centred and systematic assessment of physical, emotional, psychological, social cultural and spiritual needs, including risk, and together, develops a comprehensive personalised plan of nursing care.

10. People can trust the newly registered graduate nurse to deliver nursing interventions and evaluate their effectiveness against the agreed assessment and care plan.

*By entry to the register:*

x.  Involves the person in review and adjustments to their care, communicating these changes to colleagues.

## Chapter aims

By the end of this chapter, you should be able to:

*   understand, explain and apply systematic clinical decision-making;
*   describe the use of systematic decision-making in the nursing process;
*   apply the nursing process in systematically assessing the activities of living;
*   apply systematic clinical decision-making in evidence-based practice.

# Introduction

So far, in our exploration of clinical judgement and decision-making we have looked at nursing concepts (Chapter 1), collaborating with patients/families and healthcare teams (Chapter 2), and using observation skills to inform decisions (Chapter 3). This chapter combines and applies the different strands from earlier chapters within **systematic clinical decision-making**, a methodical, disciplined and comprehensive approach to patient-centred nursing and healthcare.

The term 'systematic' means *making use of, or carried out according to, a clearly worked-out plan or method* (Chambers, 2010). A helpful method that we can apply to any situation of working out what has happened and what to do about it is to ask the right sequence of questions, as identified in the following extract of a poem by Rudyard Kipling:

> *I keep six honest serving men*
> *(They taught me all I knew)*
> *Their names are What and Why and When*
> *And How and Where and Who*
> (Kipling, 1902)

The five 'W' questions (Who/What/Where/When/Why) can be related to Chapters 1–3, while the 'H' question (How) is the main focus of clinical decision-making in this chapter, as follows.

Clinical judgement and decision-making in nursing

| | |
|---|---|
| Who *does it involve?* | *Collaborative (Chapter 2)* |

| | |
|---|---|
| What *is the problem?* | |
| Where *does it occur?* | *Observation (Chapter 3)* |
| When *does it occur?* | |

| | |
|---|---|
| Why *make a decision?* | *Nursing theory (Chapter 1)* |
| How *to make decisions?* | *Systematic (Chapter 4)* |

This relatively simple yet effective system of questions can be applied to reflect on situations we encounter and decisions we make in our professional development as nurses (Jasper, 2006). It can also help us to examine and integrate each stage of the decision-making process in nursing.

This chapter begins by clarifying what systematic clinical decision-making means, then explains and illustrates its use: a) in a problem-solving nursing process; b) in addressing needs identified in the activities of living model; and c) in delivering sound, evidence-based, patient-centred care. Finally, the strengths and weaknesses of systematic clinical decision-making are summarised.

Activity 4.1 asks you to reflect on what was said in this chapter's introduction, and then apply Kipling's questions to review a decision you have taken.

---

## Activity 4.1                                    *Decision-making*

Given that the nurse's everyday decisions directly affect the lives of patients in their care, for the purposes of this activity try to identify and reflect on a decision you took regarding a significant event in your own life – for example, deciding to study nursing. Please apply Kipling's six questions to explore the decision-making process you went through. You might ask the following questions.

WHO?    Who did you consult before making a decision? Who else has been affected by it? Has the decision helped or hindered you in being who you want to be?

WHAT?    What made you commit three years of your life to study nursing? What might motivate or demotivate you to complete the programme?

WHERE?    Where did you live before and after starting the programme? Where else could you have studied? What made you opt to study nursing where you are now?

WHEN?    When you made your decision, what was happening in your life? What makes this the right time to study nursing?

WHY?    Why did you decide to study nursing? Why did you not choose other health-care professions or non-health related jobs?

*continued opposite . . .*

*continued . . .*

> HOW? How did you hear about studying nursing? How did you prepare yourself for the selection interview? How have you adapted your lifestyle to be a student nurse?
>
> After answering these questions in relation to a significant personal decision, write down how you think each of the six questions may help nurses to assess patients' health problems.
>
> *Some possible answers to the last question can be found at the end of the chapter.*

Working through Activity 4.1 and applying the six questions to an event with which you are personally familiar should have helped you appreciate their potential usefulness in uncovering underlying factors that uniquely influence each judgement and decision in pursuing your life goals. Similarly, in applying the six questions to assess health problems you have a practical tool to understand the unique way each individual patient experiences, and is affected by, ill health. In order to relate this way of asking questions to nurses' systematic clinical decision-making we need to find out more about the required skills and how to apply them.

# What is systematic clinical decision-making?

Like other decision-making skills discussed in this book, systematic decisions were identified by researching nursing students' experience and understanding of their development in becoming registered nurses (Standing, 2005). In the case study below, Jo, a nursing student, is asked to imagine that she is a patient and say what sort of nurse she would like to have.

## Case study: Imagining oneself as a patient

*Jo was asked about the qualities and skills she would value in a nurse if she was a patient (service user) needing care and attention. She replied:*

*'I want a nurse who is always thinking about what they are doing and why they are doing it. If I am prescribed medication, I don't want a nurse to simply give the drug because the doctor says so; I want a nurse who is going to think "Why does this person need this drug? Is it the correct dose? In what form should it be given? When should it be given? What potential unwanted side effects from the drug may occur?" If I have to have an operation, I want a nurse who is going to think "Is that really the best dressing to put on the wound?" If I happen to have burnt both my hands, I don't want a nurse in such a hurry to feed me it feels like the food is being "shovelled" into my mouth; I want a nurse who engages with me and is considerate of my preferred way of eating and drinking.'*

In the case study, Jo illustrates how asking Who/What/Where/When/Why/How questions can make a useful contribution to systematic clinical judgement and decision-making (which is characterised by combining critical thinking and problem-solving skills in giving patient-centred nursing care). For the purposes of this book the meaning of these terms is taken as follows:

*Critical thinking – purposefully question the basis of own and others' assumptions, address gaps in knowledge, challenge illogical or unethical beliefs or practice, evaluate strength of available evidence, and an ability to make a logical evidence-based argument and defend it if challenged.*

*Problem solving – dissatisfaction with a current situation prompts use of critical thinking skills to identify and assess problem, plan and implement action to remedy it, and check if it worked.*

*Systematic clinical decisions – use of critical thinking and problem-solving skills to identify/assess patient's problem, set goals/make plans, deliver care and evaluate outcome (revise as needed).*

In Table 4.1 Jo's use of critical thinking is related to Bloom's (1956) range of cognitive ability.

| Level | Critical thinking | Jo's examples |
|---|---|---|
| 1 | *Knowledge* (remember things) | Know about – medication, its correct dose and purpose; types of wound dressings; care of burns; principles of feeding patients. |
| 2 | *Comprehension* (understand things) | Understand implications of knowledge e.g. how medicine helps relieve patients' symptoms or why unwanted side effects occur. |
| 3 | *Application* (do things) | Use knowledge/understanding to assess needs and inform care. |
| 4 | *Analysis* (examine things) | Question plan of care and the roles and responsibilities of nurse, patient, doctor in its formulation and implementation. |
| 5 | *Synthesis* (create things) | Combine knowledge, skills, attitudes to ensure care has sound rationale, is technically competent, and is sensitively delivered (empathise with and help burns victim unable to feed himself) |
| 6 | *Evaluation* (critique things) | Review nursing interventions and outcomes of care and modify care plan if needed e.g. consider an alternative wound dressing. |

*Table 4.1 Different levels of critical thinking skills in systematic decision-making*

Level 1 (knowledge) is the simplest and Level 6 (evaluation) is the most complex critical thinking skill in systematic decision-making. Knowledge and comprehension (Levels 1–2) relate to theoretical understanding. Application and analysis (Levels 3–4) are where theory is applied to practice in the delivery of nursing care. Synthesis and evaluation (Levels 5–6) show a high degree of integration of theory and practice, each of which influences the other. Jo's examples (in which she alludes to the five 'Ws' and 'H' questions) relate to the whole range of critical thinking skills. Synthesis and evaluation are key graduate skills that are needed to enable nurses to make complex clinical judgements and decisions. Hence critical thinking skills are now seen as vital elements in effective problem solving and systematic clinical decision-making by nurses. Activity 4.2 asks you to relate critical thinking to your own 'patient' view of nursing.

---

### Activity 4.2                                   *Reflection and critical thinking*

Take a moment to reflect on Jo's view of nursing from a patient's perspective. Imagine you are a patient and write down what you would value about the qualities and skills of the nurses. Think of some examples and match them to the different levels of critical thinking in Table 4.1. Notice whether there are aspects of problem solving and systematic decision-making in your examples. You may want to compare notes with some of your colleagues to see how much you agree or disagree with each other.

*As this is for your own reflection, no outline answer is given.*

---

Activity 4.2 reminds us that combining critical thinking and problem-solving skills in systematic clinical decision-making is of little value unless it is patient-centred, effectively addressing their needs and preferences. In the next section we look at how the nursing process revolutionised systematic problem solving.

# The nursing process and systematic decision-making

The nursing process was developed in the USA in the 1970s, applying scientific methods within a systematic and continuous cycle of problem solving, to guide individualised nursing care. In the early 1980s the introduction of the nursing process in the UK can be likened to the policy (and impact) of evidence-based practice in twenty-first-century healthcare. Both the nursing process and evidence-based practice offer a means to apply theory to practice in a logical, organised and systematic way to improve the quality of care, and effectively address patients' needs, health problems and preferences. Figure 4.1 identifies the key stages in the nursing process, summarises their specific function in problem solving, and illustrates the process's ongoing cyclical nature (adapted from an original description by Yura and Walsh, 1973). As such, it provides a useful structure with which to understand and apply the principles of systematic clinical decision-making in nursing.

The stages shown in Figure 4.1 broadly correspond to Peplau's theory of interpersonal relations in mental health nursing (Chapter 1), but with more emphasis on problem solving and less on relationship building. In addition, the nursing process can be applied in any field of healthcare.

- Assessment (and reassessment) of patients' health problems and care needs

  ↓

- Planning strategies to address the identified health problems and care needs

  ↓

- Implementing agreed nursing interventions in delivering individualised care

  ↓

- Evaluation of care outcomes to see if problems have been resolved or not

*Figure 4.1: Nursing process*

It represents a very significant development in the professional identity of nurses, as it provided us with the tools to independently and systematically assess patients' needs and plan, deliver and evaluate care. Applying the nursing process effectively enables nurses to be autonomous health professionals. The case study below illustrates systematic clinical decision-making using the nursing process.

## Case study: Using who, what, where, when, why and how questions

*Michelle, a second-year student on placement in a children's hospital unit, is asked by her mentor to admit Annie and her three-month-old son Eric, and carry out an assessment. Michelle uses the five 'Ws' and 'H' questions (Who has, what is, where and when it is, and why and how it is a problem) when asking Annie to explain her concerns about Eric.*

*WHO?*  Eric has a feeding problem and Annie has become sore from breastfeeding him.

*WHAT?*  Eric is vomiting after feeding, he always seems hungry and he is not gaining weight.

*WHERE?*  Usually at home but also when visiting family – anywhere, in fact, if he has had a feed.

*WHEN?*  Soon after feeding. It has been getting progressively worse over the last few weeks.

*WHY?*  Annie has breastfed Eric so tried baby formula bottle milk instead to see if it made a difference, but it did not. She even tried different brands of baby milk, but Eric continued to vomit. She is worried that Eric is not going to survive if something is not done to keep his feed down.

*HOW?*  Sometimes it is 'like a white fountain shooting out of his mouth' (projectile vomiting) and after being sick Eric wants to feed again straightaway. Michelle asks Annie if she can watch the next time she feeds Eric. Annie breastfeeds Eric, and shortly after he vomits back the milk.

*Michelle discusses the assessment with her mentor, who asks her to accompany Annie and Eric to Radiology for an ultrasound examination of Eric's stomach. The results show he has pyloric stenosis (narrowing of the passage between the stomach and small intestine caused by build-up of muscle) preventing sufficient food from*

*continued opposite . . .*

*continued . . .*

*being absorbed. The medical diagnosis explains Eric's symptoms and he is scheduled for keyhole surgery (laparoscopic pyloromyotomy) the next day to remove excess muscle. The nursing care plan includes pre- and post-operative care of Eric, monitoring the intravenous line (inserted by a doctor) and fluids, checking and cleaning the wound near his belly button, and reintroducing milk feeds the day after surgery. Michelle also asks her mentor if she can give Annie some Vaseline to heal sores before she breastfeeds again as she was so concerned about Eric that she forgot to bring some for herself. Annie is relieved that they know what the problem is, that she is not to blame in any way and was right to seek help, and that the operation usually completely cures the problem. She also appreciates Michelle's concern for her. A day after surgery Eric feeds without vomiting and the next day Annie takes him home.*

Eric's condition required surgical intervention to cure it, but resolving his problem also depended on the nursing care he and his mother received. By applying the five 'Ws' and 'H' questions in the assessment, Michelle gained an understanding not only of the main health problem (Eric vomits after feeding) but also how it was affecting both Eric (always hungry, not gaining weight) and Annie (fearful about Eric dying, anxious to know what the problem is, feeling guilty that she might be at fault, and sore from breastfeeding a baby who is never satisfied). Hence, care delivery depended on collaboration (Chapter 2) and observation (Chapter 3) as nurses complemented the surgical team by controlling pre-operative risks (ensure Eric is clean, well hydrated from intravenous fluids, nil by mouth so stomach empty to prevent inhalation of vomit during surgery) and post-operative risks (risk of post-anaesthetic vomiting, ensure airway kept clear, prevent infection of wound and intravenous line). The nurses also closely collaborated with Annie in enabling her to understand what was wrong with Eric, being supportive in understanding her concerns, and helping to relieve her soreness. This was necessary for Annie to be physically and psychologically refreshed and ready to care for Eric, including gradually resuming feeding him the day after his operation. This helped to ensure that the most important collaborative relationship – bonding between mother and baby – was enhanced by the experience they shared in hospital, which was vital for Eric's future healthy development.

The case study shows how the nursing process can guide nurses' systematic clinical judgement and decision-making in assessment, planning, delivery and evaluation of care. It also illustrates how using the nursing process enables us to complement the roles of other health professionals (e.g. the surgical team) while ensuring care is tailored to the individual needs of patients and their families. Our chances of success in achieving both these aims is increased by continually using the five 'Ws' and 'H' questions to identify and review not just health problems but also how they affect the individuals concerned. Questioning develops our critical thinking (know, understand, do, examine, create and critique), which helps us to integrate problem-solving and patient-centred care in systematic clinical judgement decision-making. Activity 4.3 asks you to use your critical thinking skills to review how the nursing process is applied in practice.

**Activity 4.3**  *Decision-making and critical thinking*

Each clinical practice setting often looks after patients with similar healthcare problems, which can result in similarities in the systematic assessment, planning and delivery of nursing care. The aim of this activity is for you to compare and contrast care plans for patients with similar conditions in order to see whether there is any variation in the care plans, and if they do vary, whether it reflects patients' different individual circumstances or some other reason. If care is truly patient-centred, we would expect some variation in care plans, and if there is little difference between them, it suggests they could be tailored better to each patient's unique situation. Suppose your mentor asks you to propose a way of making the care plans more patient-centred. What strategies can you suggest for making nursing care plans more relevant and responsive to patients' individual differences?

*Some possible answers can be found at the end of the chapter.*

Activity 4.3 assumes you will find that the nursing process is still widely used in clinical practice to guide the systematic assessment, planning, delivery and evaluation of care. The process also encourages nurses to keep accurate records, which aids communication in the healthcare team and provides evidence of clinical judgements, decisions and actions for which they are accountable. The continuing relevance of the nursing process is evident in the standards for pre-registration nursing education (NMC, 2010a) – see the boxes at the start of this chapter – and in the International Council of Nurses competency framework for post-registration specialist nurses (ICN, 2009).

Some have criticised the focus on problem solving in the nursing process as being too much like a medical model and not capturing the uniqueness of nursing (Parse, 1992) or so standardised that individualised care is overlooked (Benner, 1984). Others argue that the nursing process ought to be supplemented by critical thinking skills (Corcoran-Perry and Narayan, 1995; Alfaro-LeFevre, 2009) and used in tandem with more comprehensive nursing theories/models (Griffith and Christensen, 1982). In completing Activity 4.3 you were faced with some of these issues and asked to work out a solution. In the next section we explore how combining the nursing process with the activities of a living model can help relate theory to practice in individualising systematic clinical decision-making.

# Activities of living and systematic decision-making

In the case study on pages 58–9 we saw how the nursing process guides systematic decision-making in identifying a problem and contributing to its resolution (Eric's digestion of food and fluids was compromised by an abnormality in his stomach requiring surgical correction). Eating and drinking is one of 12 activities of living described by Roper et al. (2000) that we engage in to satisfy physical, psychological and social needs – see Table 4.2. Activities of living prioritised in caring for Eric were breathing (risk of inhaling vomit), maintaining safe environment (unable to protect himself) and personal cleansing and dressing (risk of infection). The activities of the living model is, therefore, helpful in directing our attention to problems patients may have and in understanding *why* this threatens their health and well-being. It is a valuable theoretical framework to combine with the nursing process in applying systematic clinical decision-making in individualised, patient-centred care. Table 4.2 applies the concepts of *human being, environment, health* and *nurse's role and decision-making* used in Chapter 1 (Table 1.1) to the activities of the living model. Each activity of living is influenced by physical, psychological, 'sociocultural' (including spiritual), environmental, and 'politicoeconomic' (including legal) factors. Furthermore, a person's ability to carry out these activities varies from complete independence to complete dependence upon others in relation to health status, stage of development in lifespan and individual choice.

| **Human being** | **Environment** | **Health** | **Nurse's role and decision-making** |
|---|---|---|---|
| Have bio-psycho-social-spiritual needs individually met via activities of living: <br> *Maintaining a safe environment* <br> *Communicating* <br> *Breathing* <br> *Eating and drinking* <br> *Eliminating* <br> *Cleansing and dressing* <br> *Controlling body temperature* <br> *Mobilising* <br> *Working and playing* <br> *Expressing sexuality* <br> *Sleeping* <br> *Dying* | *Physical*: source of air, water, food, warmth, shelter, modes of transport <br><br> *Sociocultural*: roles, relationships and ethical or spiritual beliefs and values shaped by culture <br><br> *Politicoeconomic*: legislation controls the distribution of healthcare funding and resources | *Health*: associated with independence of individuals in carrying out their activities of living during lifespan as befits their age (dependent baby is usually healthy) <br><br> *Ill health*: physical or psychological, associated with more dependence on others in one's activities of living | Give individualised, systematic care by: <br><br> collaborating with patients (and others) to *assess* their level of independence and dependence in the activities of living; <br><br> setting goals, *planning* care to complement and/or supplementing patients' ability to carry out activities of living; *implementing* interventions; and, *evaluating* outcomes. |

*Table 4.2: Activities of living model (Roper et al., 2000) and systematic decision-making*

The 12 activities of living listed in Table 4.2 apply to all of us as human beings, and the way we carry them out is affected by environmental factors and our individual (physical and psychological) differences and preferences. They offer us, as nurses, a comprehensive and practical guide to understanding each patient as a unique individual while identifying activities of living they are having problems with that require our help. It incorporates the nursing process to guide our systematic clinical judgement and decision-making in individualised care according to problems identified during assessment and the priorities and goals of the resulting care plans. In this way they help us to look beyond a medical condition or illness, and gain a more holistic understanding of how health problems impact on individual patients and their families.

Some of the activities of living, such as breathing and eating and drinking, appear to have more immediate relevance to our health and sense of well-being. The relevance of others, such as communicating, may be less obvious, but the case study illustrated its importance as Eric was unable to tell anyone what was wrong with him, and without his mother advocating on his behalf he would not have received vital medical and nursing care. 'Expressing sexuality' may, at first glance, seem a strange one to consider in a nursing assessment, but we cannot treat people as individuals without acknowledging their sexuality, and in some situations this is related to specific health problems. Even Eric's medical problem (infantile pyloric stenosis) is gender related as boys are four times more susceptible than girls (Hernanz-Schulman, 2003). Similarly, 'dying' is not something that immediately springs to mind when thinking about what we do every day, but we know it is inevitable, and illness, accident or conflict can threaten survival at any time. In the case study Annie's fear that Eric could die was understandable (although mortality rates are now low for pyloric stenosis). Originally it was identified only by post-mortem examination, and 100 years ago 50 per cent of babies with the condition died from it (Hernanz-Schulman, 2003).

The next case study applies the activities of living model to systematic decision-making with an adult patient who has a long-term medical condition for which there is no known cure.

## Case study: Assessing a patient's activities of living

*Serena is a student nurse at the end of her second year on placement in a medical unit. During 'handover' she hears about Charlotte, aged 47, a new admission with a medical diagnosis of multiple sclerosis (erosion of protective insulation around the myelin sheath of nerves) and a history of remissions – when she is fairly independent – and relapses – when she is highly dependent. Over the last two years the relapses have got more frequent and severe. On this occasion her partner Anita raised the alarm because she can no longer physically cope. Serena is asked by her mentor to apply the activities of living model to assess Charlotte's problems, set goals and plan care.*

*Maintaining a safe environment*    Problem*: Charlotte cannot stand or walk unassisted, has poor hand co-ordination, poor eyesight, and lacks feeling in hands and feet.* Goal*: prevent injury from falling, having accident, or scalding herself.* Plan*: closely observe/supervise all activities, review ways to lengthen remission periods with medical team e.g. treatment to boost immune system.*

*Communicating*    Problem*: Charlotte has difficulty in speaking clearly.* Goal*: to understand what Charlotte's likes and dislikes are, and help her express herself.* Plan*: allow more time for her to talk, observe body language, refer for speech and language therapy (SALT) assessment, and ask Anita for communication tips.*

*Breathing*    Problem*: when Charlotte's saliva goes down the wrong way and she has coughing fit.* Goal*: prevent choking and chest infection.* Plan*: when awake support Charlotte in sitting up so she can take deep breaths, and when asleep turn her onto her side to keep her airway clear.*

*continued opposite . . .*

*continued . . .*

*Eating and drinking*    Problem: *Charlotte has difficulty in swallowing.* Goal: *ensure adequate and safe (avoid choking) fluids and nutrition.* Plan: *fluid chart, minimum 2 litres daily, check weight, refer to dietician and SALT team, give non-spill easy-to-hold cup, assist Charlotte to feed herself.*

*Eliminating*    Problem: *Charlotte has poor bladder control, smelly urine and constipation.* Goal: *prevent urinary incontinence and infection, and relieve constipation.* Plan: *send urine sample for analysis, record output on fluid chart, two-hourly toileting, high fibre supplements and laxatives.*

*Personal cleansing/dressing*    Problem: *Charlotte cannot bathe herself, and dresses/undresses with difficulty.* Goal: *good personal hygiene and well attired.* Plan: *enable Charlotte to wash hands/face, give daily 'sit in' bath/shower, and ask Anita to bring loose, comfortable clothes.*

*Controlling body temperature*    Problem: *Charlotte's hands and feet are often cold to touch.* Goal: *prevent hands and feet from getting cold.* Plan: *ask Anita for warm socks and mittens, encourage Charlotte to wriggle toes and rub hands together, and inform medical team about it.*

*Mobilising*    Problem: *Charlotte is immobile, has spasms and stiffness in legs; skin lacks elasticity, and she is at risk of getting pressure sores.* Goal: *prevent pressure sores and muscle wasting, and relieve stiffness.* Plan: *assess and monitor pressure area risks using Waterlow scale, provide pressure relief mattress/seat cushion, change position every two hours, encourage passive limb movement, refer to physiotherapy, give prescribed medication (corticosteroids), ask medical team about research supporting use of cannabis to treat spasms/stiffness, use approved lifting techniques and equipment (slide sheets, hoist), and co-ordinate teamwork to change her position or move her from bed to chair safely (without scraping her skin, alarming her or injuring nurses).*

*Working and playing*    Problem: *when in remission Charlotte volunteers in a charity shop, she used to enjoy reading before sight deteriorated, and she likes classical music.* Goal: *enable Charlotte to experience things that she enjoys.* Plan: *check with medical team whether sight can be improved, check library service for talking books or music she might like to listen to.*

*Expressing sexuality*    Problem: *Charlotte is upset by physical deterioration and feels unattractive.* Goal: *support Charlotte in recognising her attractive qualities.* Plan: *acknowledge Charlotte's achievements in doing what she can for herself, refer to beautician to manicure nails, encourage her to comb or brush hair before Anita visits, and make positive remarks about her appearance.*

*Sleeping*    Problem: *Charlotte's sleep could be disturbed due to her being turned regularly.* Goal: *minimise sleep disturbance when turning her.* Plan: *explain nurses will carefully turn her from side to side every two hours and why it is important (so she is not taken too much by surprise if she wakes up), and ask Charlotte if she would like the doctor to prescribe sleeping tablets.*

*Dying*    Problem: *Charlotte is frightened about dying.* Goal: *give Charlotte accurate information about her illness, treatment and expected outcomes in a supportive manner.* Plan: *ask doctor to explain Charlotte's prognosis regarding her current relapse and future life expectancy, ask Charlotte if she would like Anita to be present when the doctor talks to her, and ensure that Charlotte and Anita have details of the Multiple Sclerosis Society where they can get more information and support.*

The case study illustrates how the activities of living model complements the nursing process in directing systematic clinical judgement and decision-making in comprehensive assessment and care planning. The focus on activities of living helps us to recognise that our role complements and supplements patients' own abilities and their level of dependence or independence. It offers an accessible structure to address a wide range of bio–psycho–social–spiritual health issues specifically tailored to each patient's unique circumstances. It also indicates how complex nursing decisions can be, while reinforcing the value of observation and collaboration with patients, families/carers and the inter-professional healthcare team. Activity 4.4 asks you to apply the activities of living model to your own clinical practice before we look at systematic clinical decision-making in evidence-based practice.

---

### Activity 4.4         *Decision-making*

Practice applying the 12 activities of living in Table 4.2 (examples are given in the case study) and apply them to systematically assess problems, set goals, and plan care for patients you have cared for in the past or you are currently caring for. Discuss your care plan with your mentor.

*As this is for you to consolidate learning in relating it to your experience, there is no outline answer.*

---

# Systematic clinical decision-making in evidence-based practice

The case studies we have looked at so far are forms of evidence because they are based on real people, events and nursing interventions that have been examined and discussed by applying relevant theory and research. In the final case study we go one step further in enabling service users themselves to learn and apply a well-researched and respected therapy as the 'primary practitioner' in highly systematic, evidence-based self-care, while the nurse adopts a collaborative, educative and supportive role. We are going to be looking at the application of cognitive behaviour therapy (CBT) by someone with anxiety and panic attacks. It is the method of choice for anxiety in the National Institute for Health and Clinical Excellence clinical guidelines (NICE, 2011). Trower et al. (1988) summarise the main principles of CBT as follows.

1. Human emotions and behaviour are prompted by thinking.
2. Negative unrealistic thinking leads to emotional disorder.
3. Stop unrealistic thinking to reduce emotional disturbance.

## Applying CBT principles in service users' self-care

Teach service users to treat themselves by being able to:

A   monitor their emotional responses and behaviour;
B   identify trigger events associated with A;

C    identify related unhelpful beliefs and thoughts;

D    make connections between thinking, emotions and behaviour;

E    examine evidence for and against unhelpful beliefs;

F    replace unhelpful thoughts with realistic helpful thoughts.

   (adapted from Trower et al., 1988)

The following case study shows how a nurse therapist is teaching a client to apply CBT to help her deal with her anxiety and panic attacks. She has set the client homework in using an ABC framework where A = activating event associated with anxiety, B = beliefs about the event (differentiate between helpful and unhelpful thoughts and images), and C = consequences of beliefs about the events (differentiate between helpful and unhelpful emotions and behaviour), the aim being to empower the client to recognise how her overly negative self-critical thoughts can make her feel bad, and to replace these with self-affirming thoughts that accurately reflect her positive characteristics (not usually acknowledged) in order for her to feel less anxious.

## Case study: Self-care using CBT to challenge self-denigrating beliefs

*Kim is a third-year student on placement in a community mental health team. She accompanies one of the nurses, Rita, a qualified cognitive behaviour therapist, to visit Carol, aged 34, referred by her GP as she gets panic attacks and is frightened of going out. Carol was divorced seven years ago, lives with daughter Judy, aged 11, and works as an assistant librarian. Last month she had to take Judy to visit her new school. Carol was very nervous about going and when she got there had a severe panic attack (heart thumping, sweaty, dizzy, felt sick and desperate for toilet). Since then she only feels safe when at home, has had time off work, will not go shopping unless Judy is with her and is very reluctant to go out anywhere. Rita saw Carol twice last week to do an initial assessment, explain how Carol could apply CBT to deal with problems, and explore what happened, how she felt, and what she was thinking at the school.*

*Rita begins by checking that Carol remembers her saying she would have a student this week and explains Kim is there to observe. She asks Carol how she feels about this. Carol says it is not a problem and she is happy for Kim to observe. Rita asks Carol if she can apply CBT to look at her decision-making in her acceptance of Kim. Carol responds by getting out one of the blank 'ABC' forms Rita gave her, and puts 'happy for Kim to observe' under C (consequences) – helpful emotions/behaviours. She puts 'Kim turning up with Rita' under A (activating event). Rita confirms that Carol correctly identified the event that triggered her decision-making and the outcome. She is aware that Carol has not identified her beliefs and asks Carol if the event itself was sufficient to bring about the outcome or if something else was needed. Carol says she knows she has to put something under B but cannot think what it is. Rita asks Carol again to at look at whether A is sufficient to explain C and she says, 'Well, we all have to learn don't we? I remember having to shadow the librarian.' 'Ah,' Rita says. 'I think you have just identified a belief about A.' Carol writes 'We all have to learn' under B (beliefs) – helpful thoughts/images. Rita asks Carol if there is anything about Kim's behaviour that might have contributed to her decision, and she says, 'Well, she seems to be taking it all in and is used to seeing mad people like me.' Rita suggests Carol puts the first part of her answer under B (beliefs) – helpful thoughts/ images – and asks her where she thinks the second part ('she is used to seeing mad people like me') should go. Carol pauses then puts it under B (beliefs) – unhelpful thoughts/images. Rita asks Carol to read out the completed*

*continued overleaf . . .*

*continued . . .*

*ABC form and explain it to Kim. Carol tells Kim it helps her to understand that it is how she makes sense of events that determines how she feels or behaves, rather than the events themselves, so she is more in control and also has an opportunity to change from unhelpful to helpful beliefs, which makes her feel more confident. A summary of this brief exchange in the ABC format Carol has learnt to apply to herself follows.*

## Carol's self-completed 'ABC' form applying CBT

| 'A' Activating event describe experience | 'B' Beliefs (about 'A') thoughts/images | 'C' Consequences (of 'B') emotions/behaviour |
|---|---|---|
| Rita (nurse therapist) arrives with Kim (nursing student) | Helpful: we all have to learn; it is like when I had to shadow the librarian at work. She (Kim) seems to be 'taking it all in'. | Helpful: It is not a problem. I am happy for Kim to observe. I feel I am doing something useful in helping Kim to learn. |
| | Unhelpful: Kim is used to seeing mad people like me. | Unhelpful: self 'put down' 'takes the shine off' my efforts to feel more self-confident. |

*Rita points out that Carol's beliefs in this instance concern Kim, and she has a golden opportunity to test the evidence (her assumptions about Kim) by checking with Kim. Kim agrees she is there to learn, that she has learnt stuff she did not know before from both of them, and that she does not think Carol is mad. Rita suggests that Kim has played her part in supporting the evidence for Carol's helpful beliefs while helping her to challenge her unhelpful beliefs, and although Carol may have said it in jest, it revealed her self-denigration, and the consequences of it can add to her anxiety, panic attacks and fear of going out. Rita sets Carol homework to complete an 'ABC' form focusing on her fear of going to the surgery, which she will explore with her next time.*

The case study shows how evidence-based CBT can be applied in community mental health care. It complements observation of physical factors, mood, thoughts and behaviour in assessing mental health (Chapter 3), and the Who/What/Where/ When/Why/How questions discussed earlier. The nurse therapist was skilful in enabling the client to apply CBT to explore her reaction to the nursing student observing her, a potentially anxiety inducing event. The student also made a positive contribution by giving feedback about the accuracies and inaccuracies of the client's assumptions about her. This provided evidence to support Carol's helpful, realistic beliefs while challenging her unhelpful, unrealistic beliefs. She also seemed to gain confidence in using the 'ABC' structure for self-assessment. Table 4.3 relates Rita and Kim's systematic decision-making in enabling Carol's self-care using CBT to conceptions of nursing. After looking at Table 4.3, see if you can apply CBT to your own experience in Activity 4.5.

| Conceptions of nursing | Systematic clinical decision-making |
|---|---|
| Caring | Support and validate Carol's ability to help herself. |
| Listening and being there | Be alert to negative beliefs Carol expresses about herself. |
| Practical procedures | Conduct interview, set new homework, arrange next visit. |
| Knowledge and understanding | Use principles of CBT for anxiety/panic attacks/low self-esteem. |
| Communicating | Question Carol about thoughts/feelings, use of CBT; give feedback to support helpful/challenge unhelpful thoughts. |
| Patience | Give Carol time to categorise and record thoughts/feelings. |
| Teamwork | Kim complemented Rita by helping Carol test assumptions. |
| Paperwork and electronic record | Give Carol 'ABC' forms so she can examine and record events, beliefs triggered by them and how they affect her. |
| Empathising and non-judgemental | Understand Carol might be anxious about Kim's presence. |
| Professional | Apply evidence-based, NICE approved, CBT interventions. |

*Table 4.3: Integrating systematic clinical decision-making with conceptions of nursing*

---

**Activity 4.5**                    *Evidence-based practice and research*

Try to complete the following mini 'ABC' form (adapted from Trower et al. 1988) to test the theory that it is our interpretations of events that determine our emotions and behaviour and not the events themselves. It might be easier to start with 'C' as emotions are vivid/easier to recall, e.g. *How* embarrassed do you feel/avoiding certain situations? 'A' *What* events do you relate to that feeling? 'B' *What* do you think about the experience and *why* do you continue to feel the way you do?

| 'A' Activating event describe experience | 'B' Beliefs (about 'A') thoughts/images | 'C' Consequences (of 'B') emotions/behaviour |
|---|---|---|
| | Helpful: | Helpful: |
| | Unhelpful: | Unhelpful: |

*As this activity is for your own personal research there is no answer provided.*

Activity 4.5 can help us to understand how events can trigger thoughts which determine how we feel and behave. This is important because unless we are able to separate and examine these different elements, then we might remain unaware of our reasoning behind decisions – and our beliefs may be mistaken. The use of CBT to examine how well our decisions match up to the available evidence encourages us to be more aware of our own biases and 'blind spots' (see also reflexivity in Chapter 8). It also complements critical thinking ability, which is a vital aspect of effective systematic clinical decision-making. In Chapter 5 we will look in more detail at evidence-based practice in relation to standardised policies, procedures and clinical guidelines.

## Chapter summary

This chapter defined and explored systematic clinical decision-making in relation to asking Who/What/Where/When/Why/How questions, enabling nurses to apply critical thinking and problem solving with patients to address their needs. We incorporated this questioning approach in applying the nursing process, an influential framework supporting systematic clinical decision-making. We saw that the nursing process needs to be supplemented by other theories to guide more comprehensive assessment/care planning and the activities of living model was shown to marry very well with it. We noted along the way that our professional practice is enhanced by being aware of relevant research evidence. We then explored how to encourage service users/patients to learn how to question the basis of their own assumptions, especially where this led to emotional or behavioural problems, and saw how changes could be made by challenging overly negative and unrealistic belief systems. This offers great potential in empowering service users, but also in enabling nurses to apply critical thinking skills in systematic clinical decision-making.

## Activities: brief outline answers

### Activity 4.1 Decision-making (pages 54–5)

You may have included some of the following points.

| | |
|---|---|
| WHO? | Who is the patient? Who are their significant others? If infectious, who have they had contact with? Who else needs to be involved in their care? |
| WHAT? | What has made the patient seek help? What aspects of their bio–psycho–social–spiritual needs do they have difficulty with? What are their most urgent needs? |
| WHERE? | If in pain, where does it hurt? If in an accident, where did it happen? If a psychological problem, which social or environmental settings make it better or worse? |
| WHEN? | When did they first notice the problem? When does it affect them? During year/month/day/night? When doing certain activities? Are they experiencing the problem now? |
| WHY? | Why does the patient think they developed a health problem? Why are they unable to resolve it themselves? Why is nursing care needed (or not) for the patient? |
| HOW? | How has the patient's life been affected by the problem? How have they/their families/others managed to cope with it so far? How can nursing care make a difference? |

### Activity 4.3 Decision-making and critical thinking (page 60)

You may have included some of the following points.

- Incorporate who/what/where/when/why/how questions, especially when assessing/reassessing patients (see answer guide to Activity 4.1).
- As well as identifying the health problem, find out how it is affecting the patient and family, and use this knowledge to inform individualised aspects of the care plan.
- Combine systematic/collaborative/observation in decision-making so patients' needs and preferences influence care plans, which are continually evaluated and revised as needed.
- Review patients' care plans using Bloom's range of critical thinking skills (see Table 4.1) to explore ways of making them more relevant to each patient's needs.

## Further reading

**Ellis, P** (2010) *Evidence-based Practice in Nursing.* Exeter: Learning Matters. Excellent introduction to evidence-based practice for nurses.

## Useful websites

**www.mssociety.org.uk**

Award winning Multiple Sclerosis Society website packed with the latest information, research and advice for patients, carers and professionals.

# Chapter 5
# Standardised clinical decision-making

*continued . . .*

*By the first progression point:*

iii. Under supervision assesses risk within current sphere of knowledge and competence.

*By the second progression point:*

vii. Contributes to promote safety and positive risk taking.

*By entry to the register:*

xiv. Works within policies to protect self and others in all care settings including in the home care setting.

## Chapter aims

By the end of this chapter, you should be able to:

- explain standardised clinical decision-making;
- identify local policies/procedures influencing decisions;
- assess how health policy influences clinical decisions;
- apply evidence-based clinical guidelines to decisions;
- understand the pros and cons of standardised decision-making.

# Introduction

At the start of each chapter in this book (and other books in the same series) you see selected NMC standards for pre-registration nursing education and related competencies. This is an example of standardisation, which involves identifying minimum acceptable standards for any product or process and then ensuring that all examples conform to the agreed formula. Setting standards in nursing education helps prepare you in the knowledge, skills, attitudes, values and standards of professional conduct (NMC, 2008) that you need to demonstrate as a registered nurse.

Standardisation is prevalent in all walks of life; for example, you could go into any restaurant of a particular fast food chain anywhere in the world and expect to get the same meal prepared to the same standard. The formula is successful because the product is popular and keenly priced, and customers know what to expect. Getting it right requires good market research to develop appealing recipes, policies and business plans. These ensure the effective management of restaurants in sourcing, preparing and serving flavoursome meals. The same basic principles are applied in assuring the quality of good-value healthcare, which is also influenced by research evidence, national policies, standards and guidelines regarding local practice. In addition, healthcare professionals are required to follow agreed clinical procedures in order to ensure that care or treatment is safe and effective, and with a high level of patient satisfaction.

In this chapter we apply the principles of standardisation to clinical decision-making in nursing. We start by clarifying what standardisation means and then look at its application in local clinical procedures and the influence of government health policy and evidence-based clinical guidelines. Finally, the strengths and weaknesses of **standardised clinical decision-making** are summarised.

# What is standardised clinical decision-making?

Standardised clinical decision-making was identified as a significant theme when researching nursing students' perceptions, experience and development of clinical decision-making skills (Standing, 2005), as illustrated in the following case study.

## Case study: Students: perceptions of standardised decision-making

*After 18 months on a pre-registration nursing programme students were asked to describe their experience and involvement in patient care and how they perceived clinical decision-making. A number of them made similar comments about the apparent predetermined or prescribed nature of many nursing decisions, particularly in relation to assessment and planning care.*

*Some students saw standardised decision-making as a positive thing.*

- *'Luckily they use Roper's model, which I am keen on. The care plans and assessment forms are all pre-printed so you just follow a list of questions.'*
- *'The care plans are computerised and they have highly structured forms to fill in so that you cannot forget to ask about things that are relevant.'*
- *'The standardised care plans on the ward very much cover all the angles. So care planning is "covering all the bases" making sure you have an appropriate response for almost anything that might happen.'*

*Other students were less enthusiastic about standardised decision-making, as follows:*

- *'Every ward has a filing cabinet full of core care plans.'*
- *'You get a patient, you go to a drawer, and there is a numbered care plan.'*
- *'We use core care plans following the Roper model but I don't like them.'*

*(Standing, 2005, pp89–90)*

The case study suggests that the nursing process and activities of living model (Roper et al., 2000) – discussed in relation to systematic decision-making in Chapter 4 – were adopted as standardised templates to assess patients' problems or needs, and in planning care. Students who thought this was a good thing appreciated the way it helped them know what to ask patients, how to record their responses, and how this contributes to the delivery of effective patient care. For other students standardised 'core care plans' appeared part of a task-orientated routine in which they were unable to identify any specific benefits either for patients or for themselves. To optimise the benefits of standardised decision-making (e.g. not having to 'reinvent the wheel' in care plans for patients with similar problems) we need to combine it with observation, collaborative and systematic decision-making (Chapters 2–4), so that care meets patients' individual needs.

In some cases the core care plans referred to by students were not restricted to nursing as they represented the total care received by patients from all the healthcare professionals. These are examples of integrated care pathways (ICPs) that are characterised by the following features.

- Use standardised, systematic, collaborative and inter-professional care planning.
- Focus on patients who share a similar medical condition or health problem.
- Are developed, implemented and audited locally by health professionals and patients.
- Incorporate latest relevant research findings to guide evidence-based practice.
- Identify key goals on the 'patient journey' from initial assessment to discharge.
- Coordinate roles and responsibilities for care by different healthcare professionals.
- Share inter-professional documenting of care, which avoids unnecessary duplication.
- Record variation from ICP goals and explain professional judgement.
- Give patients an outline of what to expect and how they can contribute to care.
- Enhance quality of care, reducing variations in standards among practitioners.
  (Campbell et al., 1998; Middleton et al., 2001)

Standardised clinical decision-making associated with the assessment, planning, delivery and evaluation of nursing care is influenced by many factors, including the nature of patients' problems, health policy, research, local procedures, teamwork and organisation. For the purposes of this book standardised clinical decision-making is defined as follows:

> *Standardised clinical decision-making applies NHS Trust policies and procedures, agreed care plans and evidence-based guidelines/assessment tools uniformly and consistently to patient care.*

Standardised clinical decision-making in nursing was identified by students like you reflecting on their experiences, and Activity 5.1 asks you to reflect on your own observations in this respect.

---

## Activity 5.1        *Reflection*

How does your experience compare with that of students in the case study? Take a moment to think about your observations of standardised clinical decision-making regarding assessment tools, planning care, clinical procedures and guidelines applied in your practice placements. Describe an example of standardised decision-making; identify the intended benefits for patients, what the outcomes were, and what you learned about clinical decision-making. Was your example of standardised decision-making supplemented by observation, collaborative decision-making or systematic decision-making? If so, how? Why do you think this was necessary? What was the effect of doing so?

*As this is for your own reflection there is no outline answer provided.*

# Standardised decision-making in clinical procedures

So far we have ascertained that nursing education is standardised so that patients can receive safe, effective and competent care relevant to their needs, whichever registered nurse is on duty. We have looked at ways in which nurses' decision-making is standardised and how this may be complemented by observation, collaborative and systematic decision-making in tailoring care for each patient. The next case study combines these elements as a student has to demonstrate competence in a clinical procedure to pass an assessment, while also being sensitive to the patient's needs.

## Case study: Catheterising complications

*Lawrence is a registered mental health nurse doing a shortened post-registration adult nursing programme. He is on placement in an acute medical hospital ward where he is due to be assessed in carrying out a clinical procedure safely and effectively using aseptic 'non-touch' technique to avoid contaminating sterile areas. Lawrence is anxious because he is more skilled in talking to patients than he is in physical care but must pass to stay on the programme.*

*Frank, aged 68, a retired bricklayer, usually very fit, is admitted to investigate why he has been tired over the last few weeks, unable to do gardening, which he normally loves, and why he has lower back pain. Frank cannot provide a urine sample, and medical examination reveals a distended bladder from chronic urinary retention associated with an enlarged prostate gland. Frank has not told anyone he has problems urinating before. Lawrence discusses Frank's care with his mentor. The goal is for Frank to empty his bladder. The plan is to catheterise Frank. Lawrence has observed and assisted in the procedure before and agrees to be assessed by his clinical mentor in catheterising Frank. He checks the clinical procedures manual. He asks Frank if he remembers what the doctor said about his bladder problem and he replies, 'I got a blocked pipe and need a plumber!' Lawrence explains urethral catheterisation, that anaesthetic gel will be used to reduce his discomfort, and checks if Frank agrees to him carrying out the procedure with the mentor observing, which he does. Lawrence says he will be back soon and draws curtains around Frank's bed for privacy, leaving a space to come back in. Lawrence washes hands with chlorhexidine 'scrub', puts on a new disposable apron, thoroughly cleans the trolley with antiseptic, checks the contents of the sealed sterile catheter packs (male) and places one on the bottom shelf of the trolley together with other items (e.g. drainage bag, spare catheter). At the bedside Lawrence follows prescribed local aseptic procedure (e.g. wearing sterile gloves) to avoid contaminating the catheter or injuring Frank during its insertion. Before reaching the bladder, the catheter gets stuck, which gentle pressure cannot overcome so Lawrence slowly withdraws it. He explains to Frank it is best not to use force to avoid injuring him, that he could try again with a slightly larger catheter, which is more rigid and will possibly make it easier to overcome resistance. If he would rather not go through that again, an alternative type of catheter (suprapubic) could be inserted directly into the bladder by the doctors. He might find this a more comfortable option but it does require a small surgical procedure to fit it.*

*continued opposite . . .*

*continued . . .*

*Frank opts to have a suprapubic catheter inserted by the medical team and is able to empty his bladder. Although Lawrence was unsuccessful, he passes the assessment as he followed procedure, maintained aseptic 'non-touch' technique, took care not to cause injury, kept Frank fully informed, respected his freedom of choice, and was able to explain his actions. Tests show Frank has aggressive, advanced (inoperable) prostate cancer that has spread to his back bone. Three weeks later Frank dies and Lawrence helps the staff nurse perform 'last offices' cleaning and laying out his body ready for his family to see him. Lawrence feels very thankful to Frank for allowing him to try to catheterise him despite his pain, and feels it is a great shame that Frank was not able to report symptoms before as earlier intervention might have saved him.*

The case study links standards of nursing education with standardised clinical decision-making and draws parallels between the roles of student/nurse and patient. As a student there is always another assessment to pass so your career is always 'on the line' until you eventually qualify. Even when we register as nurses we have to show our knowledge and skills are up to date and we are fit to practise or we can be removed from the NMC register. The reason why standards are stringent is that, for patients, it is not just careers but often their lives that are 'on the line'. It is why risks have to be minimised, and standardised clinical decision-making is a way to achieve this. Lawrence's use of aseptic technique to catheterise Frank was unsuccessful but he followed the correct procedure (confirmed by passing his assessment) and he could transfer these skills in caring for others. It also alerted the medical team to relieve Frank's urinary retention with a suprapubic catheter in a standardised procedure that carries different risks (Ahluwalia et al., 2006).

Table 5.1 relates standardised clinical decision-making in carrying out a practical procedure to conceptions of nursing that nurses used to describe their professional identity (Standing, 2005). It shows that Lawrence managed to combine the discipline of being adept in specific technical skills with interpersonal qualities in caring for Frank. It is important to emphasise this point: standardised clinical decision-making can be perceived as an impersonal, task-orientated routine, but this is not a reason for ignoring the individuality and preferences of patients on the receiving end of such procedures. Some of the less enthusiastic attitudes expressed by nursing students towards standardised decision-making are possibly due to their difficulty in linking such uniform practices to individualised patient-centred care. Lawrence understood he had a duty to try to catheterise Frank safely and effectively. This required him to apply the prescribed aseptic procedure to reduce the risk of introducing infection. He knew his duty of care did not end there as he was also attentive and responsive to Frank's concerns. After looking at Table 5.1, you have an opportunity to relate these issues to your own experience in Activity 5.2.

| Conceptions of nursing | Standardised clinical decision-making |
|---|---|
| Caring | Taking care to minimise Frank's discomfort |
| Listening and being there | Respecting Frank's preference for 'suprapubic' catheter rather than trying a second time via the urethral route |
| Practical procedures | Demonstrating aseptic technique to insert urethral urinary catheter by following the locally approved procedure |
| Knowledge and understanding | Anatomy, physiology of male urinary system; pathology of urinary retention and prostate cancer, plus catheter care |
| Communicating | Explaining catheterisation, checking Frank understands and consents to Lawrence carrying out the procedure |
| Patience | Waiting to allow time for anaesthetic gel to take effect, not panicking or using excess force when catheter gets stuck |
| Teamwork | Alerting medical team that urethral catheter will not go in bladder |
| Paperwork and electronic record | Checking procedures manual and record events in care plan |
| Empathising and non-judgemental | Understanding that Frank was in pain and that catheterisation can be uncomfortable, and also potentially embarrassing |
| Professional | Demonstrating knowledge, skills, attitudes and clinical competence needed to pass practical assessment |

*Table 5.1: Integrating standardised clinical decision-making and conceptions of nursing*

## Activity 5.2                                                    *Decision-making*

Think about the various clinical procedures that you have observed or carried out with patients and choose one example to explore in more depth. Look at how Table 5.1 related Lawrence's attempted catheterisation of Frank to the conceptions of nursing and draw up a similar table to cross-reference your example of standardised decision-making with the conceptions of nursing. Do you find it easy or hard to mix technical and interpersonal skills in carrying out procedures? Do you think it is necessary to combine the two contrasting skills sets? What methods do you use to check what the patient is experiencing while

*continued opposite . . .*

*continued . . .*

carrying out a procedure? Has this resulted in you making any adjustments to the procedure or not? How helpful or unhelpful do you find it to map your clinical procedure against the conceptions of nursing?

*As this activity is for you to relate the above discussion to your clinical experience, no outline answer is given.*

So far we have discussed standardised clinical decision-making in relation to carrying out local practical procedures and Activity 5.2 has asked you to explore your own example in this respect. We also noted that competence in clinical decision-making and nursing interventions is subject to continuous assessment in preparing you to be a registered nurse responsible for patient care. In the next section we take a look at the national picture and how governments' health policies influence standardised clinical decision-making and the structuring of healthcare services.

# Health policy and standardised clinical decision-making

Each of us has standardised rights regarding our personal freedom and protection from physical or verbal harm, and standardised responsibilities in respecting the rights of others. These are our statutory rights and obligations in legislation approved by governments in Acts of Parliament. Central government also determines health policy in the UK, which gives each person a right to National Health Service (NHS) care that is free at the point of delivery (paid for indirectly via taxation). In order to ensure public money is well spent, standards are set that hospitals and community services, and health professionals, are expected to meet. As a health professional you have a right to have a high standard of education to prepare for your role, and continuing professional development opportunities to enhance your practice. In return you have a responsibility to use effective clinical decision-making skills in high quality, evidence-based, patient-centred care.

In deciding health policy, governments make use of scientific evidence to assess the nation's health with reference to morbidity (sickness) and mortality (death) rates in the population. Under *The NHS Plan* (DH, 2000), National Service Frameworks identified standards, set health targets, and monitored progress in improving health promotion, access to services, reduced waiting times and early medical intervention. One health target was to reduce deaths from cancer in the under 75s by 20 per cent by the year 2010. The lifetime chance of having female breast cancer is estimated as 1 in 9 (Cancer Research UK, 2009) and the lifetime chance of males having prostate cancer is similar at 1 in 10 (Cancer Research UK, 2010). However, standardised screening for early detection and treatment of female breast cancer (i.e. mammography) in the UK is more advanced than screening for male prostate cancer, as Frank's case study illustrates. Mammography is associated with a sensitivity (ability to detect breast cancer) of up to 90 per cent, so it is considered cost effective for national screening. There is a prostate specific antigen (PSA) blood test (raised levels linked to prostate cancer), but it is not considered sufficiently accurate or cost-effective for routine screening of males in the UK. Early detection of prostate cancer for men such as Frank relies on them alerting health professionals as soon as they have urinary problems rather than being too embarrassed to talk about it. As nurses we need to be aware of this and offer information, advice and support to encourage men at high risk (over 65s) to discuss problems.

Sometimes standardised health screening can be perceived as counter-productive, as the next case study of a child classified as being 'overweight' helps to illustrate.

### Case study: Being told you are overweight

*In August 2010 a schoolgirl, aged 11, was weighed (49 kilograms/7 stone 12 pounds) and her height measured (1.524 metres/5 feet) at school as part of the National Child Measurement Programme (NCMP). After the local NHS sent a letter saying the result indicated she was overweight, she got very upset and her mother had difficulty getting her to eat. The aim of NCMP is to promote healthy weight for healthy living and prevent obesity, which is associated with greater health risks of diabetes, cancer, heart or liver disease (DH, 2010a). Her mother was angry that a scheme designed to promote health appeared to be actually damaging her daughter's health by encouraging her to become anorexic. The story was reported in the press with pictures of the girl who appeared to have a nice figure and did not seem overweight. It poses questions about the validity of the test and any advice given (dieting, exercise) based on the results.*

The case study helps to highlight potential problems with standardised screening tests and how these need to be taken into account when decision-making, especially with children. As adults we are also encouraged to keep within recommended weight guidelines according to how tall we are. Measures of weight and height are used to calculate and categorise our body mass index (BMI): less than 18.5 = underweight; 18.5–25 = healthy weight; 25.1–30 = overweight; and over 30 = obese (NHS, 2010). To calculate an adult BMI score: measure weight; measure height; divide weight by height; divide again by height. If we use the case study weight and height measurements and pretend they belong to an adult we get the following BMI score:

| | |
|---|---|
| Weight: | 49 kilograms |
| Height: | 1.524 metres |
| Divide weight by height: | $49 \div 1.524 = 32.15223$ |
| Divide answer by height: | $32.15223 \div 1.524 = 21.09$ |
| BMI score: | 21.09 (in healthy weight range) |

We have now established that if the schoolgirl had been an adult with exactly the same weight and height, she would have been classified as being well within the healthy weight range. She was classified as overweight because children's BMI scores are adjusted to what is considered the norm for a child of that age; because she was large for her age she was outside the expected norm and labelled overweight. If the child had been just one year older with the same measurements she would have been in the healthy weight range. Health promotion encouraging healthy weight and avoiding problems of obesity is a worthwhile aim. It makes sense to educate children to help prevent problems in adulthood, and the NCMP test may be accurate in the majority of cases. However, the case study shows us that individual variations from the norm do not always mean there is something wrong with the person, and that further refinement of the tests themselves may be needed to improve their accuracy. As nurses we need to be aware of the strengths and weaknesses of standardised tests. We also need to set an example of good health, and Activity 5.3 asks you to check your BMI in this respect.

---

### Activity 5.3         *Evidence-based practice and research*

Do you know what your BMI score is? In this activity you are asked to apply this standardised tool to assess your weight range and appreciate what it is like for patients on the receiving end of numerous tests and investigations. You can calculate your BMI either manually (with the help of a calculator) by following steps taken on the previous page or by logging on to **www.nhs.uk/Tools/Pages/Healthyweightcalculator.aspx**, which has an interactive program for you to experiment with. You still need to input your height and weight, but it does the rest, giving you a BMI score and identified weight range (healthy or otherwise). You can choose to input figures as kilograms and metres or as feet/inches and stones/pounds (a metric conversion is done to calculate the BMI score), and you can print off results as a record to compare with your future scores. When you have done this, answer the following question: What factors can you identify that affect the accuracy of the BMI score that you have calculated, and how might you optimise its accuracy?

*Some possible answers can be found at the end of the chapter.*

---

Activity 5.3 gives you a taste of what it is like to have aspects of your individuality quantified and classified according to a standardised assessment tool. As we have seen, it is important to appreciate the human stories behind statistics about our health status. The UK's coalition government (elected in 2010) appears to support this point, as it proposes to replace National Service Frameworks with an NHS Outcomes Framework promoting reforms responsive to patients' experience of healthcare and satisfaction with outcomes (DH, 2010b). The National Institute for Health and Clinical Excellence (NICE) will also be expected to develop cost-effective evidence-based clinical guidelines to make improvements in healthcare outcomes. In the next section we look at evidence-based guidelines used in standardised decision-making.

# Clinical guidelines and standardised clinical decision-making

Using standardised screening techniques to assess members of the public for potential health problems needs to be combined with effective intervention tools where required. Knowing how to do this is helped by relevant evidence-based clinical guidelines. In the UK it is estimated that 24 per cent of adults drink hazardous or harmful amounts of alcohol, and that 35 per cent of

Accident and Emergency visits, 900,000 hospital visits and 15,000 deaths each year are alcohol related. In total, alcohol problems are thought to cost the NHS £2 billion annually (NHS Information Centre, 2009). The following case study describes a student who has begun to have problems with alcohol and how standardised evidence-based clinical guidelines are applied by a nurse practitioner.

## Case study: Acknowledging problems with alcohol use

*Anne, aged 20, is a second-year student at university studying hospitality management who hopes to work in hotels around the world. During term time Anne works part-time in the student union bar, and during the vacation she works in the cocktail bar of a restaurant. Anne enjoys drinking alcohol, her favourite being a 'Cuban' cocktail of spiced rum, cola and lime juice. Over the last year Anne has increased her alcohol consumption not just when she goes out with friends but also when she is serving drinks at the bar, and when she is alone in her room.*

*Anne's use of alcohol is changing from pleasant social drinking to hazardous and potentially harmful drinking. She is warned about drinking too much by the bar manager, who notices her speech is slurred; she is late for lectures and fails assignments, gets drunk at parties, strips off clothes and kisses her friend's boyfriend. Her family are very concerned about her. Then she suffers cuts and bruises when losing control of her motorbike, crashing into a lamp post after nightclubbing. She faces prosecution for riding a motorbike while three times over the limit of permitted alcohol. Anne is seen at the Accident and Emergency centre, and is advised to attend the university medical centre to discuss further medical care and support.*

*At the university medical centre, Anne is seen by Penny, a nurse practitioner, who asks what the problem is. Anne explains about her road traffic accident, the impending prosecution, and how everything generally seems to be going 'pear shaped' in her life. Penny tells Anne she cannot change what has happened but recognising that something is 'pear shaped' is a good sign because it is a starting point in deciding what changes she would like to make in her life. Penny suggests it would be useful to assess Anne's alcohol consumption, which they can do together or Anne can do it independently if she prefers. Anne agrees to complete an Alcohol Use Disorders Identification Test (AUDIT) (Saunders et al., 1993) with Penny. There are ten questions ranging from 'How often do you have a drink containing alcohol?' to 'Has a relative or friend or a doctor or another health worker been concerned about your drinking or suggested you cut down?' Each question has a choice of answers that are scored from 0 to 4. Low total scores (e.g. up to 8 out of 40) relate to safe, sociable drinking; higher scores indicate a greater risk of drinking being hazardous and harmful to health, and very high scores (e.g. over 26 out of 40) suggest possible alcohol dependence that a person may need specialist help to deal with. Anne scores 26 out of 40 and is shocked to find that her average weekly consumption of 60 units of alcohol (1 litre of rum [40 units] plus two bottles of wine [20 units]) is three times recommended levels in females (maximum 2–3 units daily or 14–21 units weekly) for safe, sociable alcohol use.*

*Anne questions the validity of the AUDIT assessment tool so Penny explains it is research based and is endorsed by major healthcare organisations, including the World Health Organization (WHO), the NHS and NICE, as an effective predictor of alcohol disorders. Anne asks what the difference is between hazardous and harmful drinking, and alcohol dependence. Penny replies that hazardous drinking means taking risks with personal health and safety (e.g. getting drunk), while harmful drinking means that ill health or injury occurs*

*continued opposite . . .*

*continued . . .*

*(e.g. motorbike crash when over alcohol limit), and alcohol dependence means knowing excessive drinking is harmful but not being able to stop doing it. Penny tells Anne that her answers indicate she should cut down her alcohol intake because drinking at her current level is associated with a higher risk of experiencing drink-related problems. She asks Anne whether her feeling that life is going 'pear shaped' might be related to her alcohol use, and Anne agrees she tends to get into trouble when she's drunk. Penny advises Anne to aim to keep within recommended levels, for example, half a litre of rum only or two bottles of wine only in a week, so she can enjoy a drink without getting so drunk she gets into trouble. Anne says she will aim to do that and put the money she saves towards repairing her motorbike so she can sell it if she gets banned, and buy a push bike instead. Penny and Anne agree to meet up again in two weeks to review progress and see whether any further support is needed.*

The standardised AUDIT assessment tool has been validated as an accurate, cost-effective way of screening and detecting alcohol problems (Wallace, 2001). It elicits information from the patient/service user for evidence of alcohol use which is mapped against lower risk or higher risk units of alcohol consumption. This provides the basis of a 'brief intervention' where the practitioner, without judging the person, ensures they understand risks of harmful drinking, the advisability of reducing alcohol use – enabling them to make an informed choice about the need to cut down – and the possible consequences of not doing so (NICE, 2010a). In Activity 5.4 you are asked to complete an AUDIT test in order to understand what is involved.

## Activity 5.4                    *Evidence-based practice and research*

As discussed above, alcohol-related health problems are common in the UK so it is important nurses understand initial screening tests, interventions and how units of alcohol are measured. To complete this activity, log on to the NHS website at **www.nhs.uk/conditions/alcohol-misuse/pages/diagnosis.aspx** where you will find a box on the left of the screen entitled 'Drinking self assessment'. This is a version of the AUDIT assessment tool that any member of the public can use. Please click 'Start' at the bottom of the box and answer the ten questions. If you are unsure how to convert drinks into units of alcohol there is an information link in Question 2 that explains it. If you do not drink alcohol, you could 'create' a character that does and answer questions accordingly. In this version of AUDIT there are three possible outcomes: drinking within sociable limits so no need to worry; could cut down as there is a risk of developing problems; may need help to cut down as level of drinking is likely to be causing problems. It is possible to print the results if you wish. Once you have finished the self-assessment, please answer the following question. What might be the limitations of the AUDIT assessment?

*Some possible answers can be found at the end of the chapter.*

Activity 5.4 gave you an opportunity to test a standardised assessment tool used to diagnose whether a person's health is at risk from their pattern of alcohol consumption. Standardised tools can also be used to prevent healthcare professionals from harming their patients by making them more aware of risks and taking steps to control them, as the following case study illustrates.

## Case study: Surgeon introduces safety checklist

*Atul, a well-respected surgeon in America, was operating on a patient using a procedure he had done numerous times before without incident, when he accidentally cut a main artery with the scalpel, causing a massive haemorrhage. Atul and the surgical team had only a couple of minutes to save the patient's life by finding and clamping the source of the haemorrhage, replacing lost blood and body fluids, and repairing the damaged artery. They could then go on to complete the scheduled operation. The patient survived but lost the sight of one eye, which had been deprived of oxygen as a result of the haemorrhage. This incident prompted Atul to learn from it and review ways of enhancing the prevention, control and management of potential risks in surgical procedures (Gawande, 2010).*

*As well as haemorrhaging, Atul was aware of many other risks associated with surgery, including: problems with anaesthesia; infection of wound site; operating on the wrong patient; operating on the right patient but the wrong site (e.g. removing left instead of right kidney). He looked at how other professions managed everyday uncertainties and controlled risks to human safety, while performing highly complex activities. He discovered that pilots referred to checklists routinely during planned 'pause moments' to review specific aspects of aircraft safety before proceeding to the next critical stage (e.g. cabin doors closed before take-off). Atul noted that while each step seemed fairly straightforward, if overlooked it could be catastrophic. He was also intrigued by research where intensive care unit nurses were asked to prompt doctors to follow a five-step checklist of questions – such as '1. Wash hands with soap' – to prevent infection by using an aseptic technique when inserting a central line (catheter in large vein near heart). Within three months reported central line infections fell by 66 per cent and after 18 months it was estimated 1,500 lives and $175 million had been saved (Pronovost et al., 2006). Atul began to think checklists could be effective in controlling risks in operating theatres and he was asked by the WHO to lead an international team in promoting safe surgery globally.*

*Atul and his team identified three critical 'pause moments' for members of the surgical team to stop and check vital safety considerations before continuing with the next stage.*

1. *Before anaesthetic is given (e.g. check identity / surgical procedure / site / consent, fit pulse oximeter to check patient's oxygen, check allergies, check if blood loss risk > 500ml).*
2. *Before an incision is made (e.g. confirm team know each others' names / roles, action plan, availability of sterile instruments, if prophylactic antibiotics given in last 60 minutes).*
3. *Before patient leaves theatre (e.g. record procedure, nurse leads review of instruments / swab count, surgeon / anaesthetist / nurse review aloud concerns about patient recovery).*

*The above became the basis of a 19-point checklist in guidelines for safe surgery (WHO, 2009). It was trialled by surgical teams in America, Canada, England, India, Jordan, New Zealand, the Philippines and Tanzania from 2007 to 2008. Death rates and complications were compared before and after introducing the*

*continued opposite . . .*

*continued . . .*

*checklist: before (3,733 patients operated on), death rate = 1.5 per cent (56), complications = 11 per cent (410); after (3,955 patients operated on), death rate = 0.8 per cent (31), complications = 7 per cent (277) (Haynes et al., 2009). So significantly fewer people died or suffered complications (e.g. infection) after the safe surgery checklist was adopted.*

These death rates may seem to be relatively low, even before introducing the checklist, but it is estimated that 234 million surgical operations occur worldwide every year (Haynes et al., 2009) so a death rate of 1.5 per cent equates to 3,510,000 deaths and a death rate of 0.8 per cent equates to 1,872,000 deaths. It suggests that adopting the safe surgery checklist throughout the world could result in 1,638,000 (3,510,000 – 1,872,000) fewer surgery-related deaths each year. Because Atul had the humility to acknowledge his mistakes as a surgeon and his dependence on the team to ensure surgery is successful (and deal with untoward incidents), he helped to create a safer system to guide surgical procedures and manage risks associated with them. In addition, he acknowledged the vital role of theatre nurses in co-ordinating the supply and monitoring of sterile instruments and equipment to minimise risks (e.g. surgeon leaving swabs inside a patient's body). Activity 5.5 asks you to think of examples of standardised procedures used to protect patients.

## Activity 5.5                                    *Team working*

Part of the success of the safe surgery checklist in the case study is that it galvanises nurses, anaesthetists, technicians and surgeons into a team who communicate and value each other's contribution to safe and successful surgery for patients. Take a moment to think about potential risks to patients' health and safety while receiving care and treatment in clinical areas that you have worked in. What examples of standardised guidelines can you identify that are used by team members to minimise these risks and protect patients from harm? Discuss your thoughts with colleagues and your mentor.

*As this is for you to review experience, no outline answer is given.*

Much of the time nurses work as part of a healthcare team and Activity 5.5 has encouraged you to think about how different team members are influenced by the same guidelines or procedures. The application of standardised health and safety guidelines is undermined if one or more team members do not adhere to them. For example, a theatre nurse was struck off the NMC register for impairment of her fitness to practise when she was held responsible for wrongly confirming all instruments were accounted for before a patient was sewn back up. The patient had a 7-inch pair of forceps left in the abdomen and required further surgery to remove them (NMC, 2010b). This example emphasises the point made earlier that our careers as nurses are always 'on the line' because patients' lives depend on us doing our jobs competently. By following standardised, evidence-based clinical decision-making we can offer higher levels of safety in controlling risks to patients' health, and in doing so enhance our professional competence.

### Chapter summary

In this chapter we looked at standardised clinical decision-making, which involves team members uniformly and consistently following agreed practical procedures, core care plans, integrated care pathways, local and national policy, and evidence-based clinical guidelines. The strengths of standardised clinical decision-making include avoiding 'reinventing the wheel' by using an evidence-based protocol or checklist to guide and quality-assure assessment, planning and delivery of specific aspects of care, and the control of associated health risks. Weaknesses of standardised clinical decision-making include the possibility of its uncritical application in task-orientated care that does not make patient-centred adjustments for individual differences. To optimise the strengths and minimise the limitations of standardised clinical decision-making, observation, collaborative decision-making and systematic decision-making (Chapters 2–4) need to be combined with it.

## Activities: brief outline answers

### Activity 5.3 Evidence-based practice and research (page 79)

You may have included the following points.

- Accuracy of equipment (scales, tape measure/height chart).
- Use of equipment, e.g. stand up straight when measured.
- Other variables, e.g. remove heavy clothing and shoes.
- Honesty of self-reporting.
- Arithmetic skills in calculating BMI.
- Variations in body types, e.g. muscular = high BMI score.

### Activity 5.4 Evidence-based practice and research (page 81)

You may have included the following points.

- Impaired recollection of alcohol use.
- Difficulty converting different drinks into units of alcohol.
- Ineffectiveness if person is intoxicated.
- Honesty of self-reporting.
- Insufficiently motivated to change.
- Need for extra criteria to assess very high dependency.

## Further reading

**Gawande, A** (2010) *The Checklist Manifesto: How to get things right.* London: Profile Books.

An excellent read that is full of fascinating true stories, such as reviving a child who has drowned, and how standardised checklists enable us to simplify and organise complex, life-saving decisions.

## Useful websites

**www.nice.org.uk/**

National Institute for Health and Clinical Excellence website where you can search for evidence-based clinical guidelines in all aspects of nursing and healthcare.

**www.nhsdirect.nhs.uk**

NHS Direct website for any member of the public to access for information and advice including a symptom checker and the recommended actions to take.

**www.doh.gov.uk**

Department of Health website where you can look at the coalition government's planned reforms of the NHS, and access archives of previous governments' policies.

# Chapter 6
# Prioritising decisions
# in delivering care

*continued opposite . . .*

*continued* . . . •••••••••••••••••••••••••••••••••••••••••••••••••••••••••••••••••••••••

vital signs, collapse, cardiac arrest, self-harm, extremely challenging behaviour, attempted suicide.

19. People can trust the newly registered graduate nurse to work to prevent and resolve conflict and maintain a safe environment.

    *By entry to the register:*

    iii. Selects and applies appropriate strategies and techniques for conflict resolution, de-escalation and physical intervention in the management of potential violence and aggression.

## Chapter aims

By the end of this chapter, you should be able to:

*   explain prioritising in clinical decision-making;
*   outline healthcare priorities in government policy;
*   organise decision-making priorities in emergency situations;
*   outline decision-making priorities in de-escalating aggression;
*   explain decision-making priorities in long-term care.

# Introduction

If someone asks, 'What are your priorities in life?', they are trying to find out what your personal beliefs and values are regarding what you think is important, and how this influences what you choose to do. As nurses, we have to abide by professional values in *The Code: Standards of conduct, performance and ethics for nurses and midwives*, the first sentence of which says:

> *The people in your care must be able to trust you with their health and well-being.*
> (NMC, 2008, p1)

This brief, simple statement seems obvious, but important truths do not need to be complicated. It portrays a key priority of nursing care, which the remaining pages of the Code reinforce when describing professional standards nurses need to achieve in order to justify the public's trust, e.g. *provide a high standard of practice and care at all times* (NMC, 2008, p1).

This chapter explores prioritising the health and well-being of patients in relation to nurses' clinical decision-making. We start by clarifying the terminology with reference to research into nursing students' perceptions of clinical decision-making skills. Relevant healthcare policy priorities are outlined, together with their implications for nursing decisions. We then discuss clinical decision-making priorities in dealing with emergency situations, in preventing and resolving conflict and aggression in clinical areas, and in supporting long-term carers.

# Clarifying terminology

'**Prioritising**' was one of ten clinical decision-making skills identified when researching students' developmental journey from the start of their programme to their first year as registered nurses (Standing, 2005). Many of the students had worked as healthcare assistants before and recognised that some patients are less able to take care of themselves than others. They associated prioritising with assessing dependency levels and giving extra help to those who needed it most. Prioritising in decision-making was associated with life saving (nurses intervening in emergency situations) as well as with recognising environmental hazards and preventing accidents from occurring.

In order to gain the public's trust in our ability to care for their health and well-being, we need to use prioritising skills in assessing and managing risks to their personal safety. In the following case study a nursing student describes his understanding of risk assessment.

## Case study: Risk assessment and life choices

*Mark is a social science graduate who volunteered on a 'nightline' service offering support to students while at university. He recently started a pre-registration nursing programme. When Mark was asked about his understanding of decision-making, and how he goes about making personal decisions, he described his view of assessing and managing potential risks.*

*'In risk assessment I suppose the idea is you multiply how likely something is to happen by how bad it would be. It is difficult to assign values to that kind of thing, but if you go skydiving, what are the odds of something going wrong and how bad would it be? If you go to a skydiving school the odds are one in something very large that something would go wrong. On the other hand, if something does go wrong and you're a mile up, then it's likely to be pretty bad, so I don't think I'll be a skydiver! You can use the same process to assess other risks. My dad is having a bit of a 'wonder' at the moment because he's always ridden a motorbike – and he's got a really nice one – but three things have gone wrong and it's costing him so much to get it repaired. He feels guilty about having a motorbike and spending too much on it when he should just get a little car because it would be safer and it wouldn't cost so much. It's like risk assessment the other way round: you take how much pleasure something gives you, then minus how much it costs you.'*

The case study indicates that there are risks associated with many life choices we make and so it makes sense to prioritise risk assessment when deciding what we are going to do. Mark's account of risk assessment/management highlights its key features.

a) Predicting and managing uncertainty (i.e. things you cannot be totally sure about).
b) Recognising that some life choices carry more health risks than others (e.g. motorbike versus car).
c) Identifying the worst case scenario, what could go wrong (e.g. parachute fails to open).
d) Recognising risks to life, health and well-being if the worst case scenario occurs.
e) Estimating the probability that something might go wrong (e.g. relevant death rates).
f) Maximising safety to minimise harm when taking risks (e.g. training, checking equipment).

g)  Weighing up costs (e.g. health risks, financial) against benefits (e.g. freedom, fun).

h)  Being accountable for deciding whether cost outweighs benefit or benefit outweighs cost.

These principles can be applied to assess health risks in any setting. As nurses it is important for us to appreciate how much uncertainty is associated with what we do everyday. We need to 'keep on our toes' regarding potential problems (e.g. risk of cross-infection) and avoid being complacent (e.g. forgetting to wash hands with antiseptic scrub before and after attending to each patient). Benefits of being vigilant in this respect include: active promotion of health and prevention or mitigation effects of illness or injury; patients being confident in our ability to look after them properly; and increased confidence for us that we are doing everything we can to ensure safety of patients. Prioritising decisions in delivering nursing care, therefore, is closely linked with risk assessment and management. For the purposes of this chapter this definition is taken to mean:

*Prioritising in decision-making applies risk assessment and management to: the immediate care of patients with life-threatening illness or injury; addressing patients' urgent needs before less urgent needs; health promotion for vulnerable groups; and the avoidance of harm to patients in care settings.*

In Activity 6.1 you are asked to apply prioritising and risk assessment in reflecting on and exploring a pastime, activity or event that you have participated in.

---

### Activity 6.1          *Reflection*

This activity is intended to help you relate prioritising and risk assessment in decision-making to your own life experience. It also highlights aspects of health promotion in relation to healthy lifestyles and preventing accidents and injuries, which is relevant to nurses' preventative role. As nurses we focus on caring for patients, but if we do not look after ourselves, we will be less able to help others. Hence we need to think about how to enhance our health and well-being.

Think about the personal choices you make about your life, apart from choosing to study be a nurse. These could include hobbies, keeping fit, attending social events, holidays, shopping trips, or simply your usual mode of transport in getting from one place to another. Choose one that you can apply the above risk assessment features to. Go through features a) to h), relate each one to your chosen activity, and write down your responses (e.g. a) anticipated uncertainty and possible risks associated with the activity and how appealing or worrying you find this, b) how safe your chosen activity is and what alternative activities are less risky or more risky). When you have finished, try to think of at least one thing you might do to enhance your own personal health and safety, and implement this in future activities if you can.

*Some possible answers can be found at the end of the chapter to compare your responses to.*

---

So far, in clarifying the terminology we have established that prioritising in clinical decision-making is closely associated with assessing and managing health risks in individual patients, and in comparing different patients' levels of dependency. We have also looked at the importance of promoting health and preventing ill health or injury to patients and the wider public both within and beyond clinical settings. These issues are also reflected in healthcare policy.

# Healthcare policy priorities and implications

## Promoting health and preventing ill health

Promoting health and preventing ill health are clearly desirable goals in health and social policy, as unnecessary suffering is prevented. It is also more cost-effective as less money is required for expensive hospital investigations, treatment, medicine and ongoing care. Nurses traditionally have contact with patients when illness or injury has already occurred. In this case preventative care is focused on avoiding complications to facilitate a speedy recovery (secondary prevention) or limiting the severity of long-term effects (tertiary prevention). There are now increasing opportunities for us to work in community care settings where we can be involved in *primary prevention*, for example, immunising children against mumps, measles and rubella (MMR), running clinics to help people give up smoking, or offering support and guidance as needed.

Health policy in the twenty-first century has placed increasing emphasis on health promotion and illness prevention. The *NHS Plan* (DH, 2000) outlined a strategy to reduce deaths from the main causes, such as coronary heart disease or stroke and cancer. Health targets were set to increase public access to services, reduce waiting times and offer early medical intervention. This appears to have contributed to a steady decline, year by year, in the number of deaths. For example, in 1999 the total number of deaths occurring in the UK was 556,118 and by 2005 the number of deaths had fallen by around 8 per cent to 512, 692 (Office for National Statistics, 2006, pxiii). Nearly two-thirds of all deaths in 2005 were due to the same two main causes, as shown in Table 6.1.

| Underlying causes of death | Number of deaths occurring |
|---|---|
| All causes (19 causes, from infections to accidents) | 512,692 (100% of all deaths) |
| Diseases of the circulatory system (e.g. coronary heart disease or stroke) | 183,997 (35.8% of all deaths) |
| Neoplasms (i.e. all cancers) | 138,454 (27% of all deaths) |
| Diseases of the circulatory system + neoplasms | 322,451 (62.8% of all deaths) |

*Table 6.1: Main underlying causes of death in the UK in 2005*

Source: Adapted from *Mortality statistics: causes* (Office for National Statistics, 2006, p2)

Table 6.1 shows that, despite a reduction in deaths from 1999 to 2005, there was still a huge proportion of deaths due to the two main causes (coronary heart disease or stroke and cancer). Hence, there is scope to reduce the incidence of these and other causes of death via health promotion, education and preventative healthcare. Lord Darzi, a practising surgeon (and also Under Secretary of State in Gordon Brown's Labour government) led an NHS review that emphasised the need to *create an NHS that helps people to stay healthy* (DH, 2008, p2). Six priorities were set for primary care trusts (GP surgeries, health centres, practice/community nurses) to focus on.

- Tackling obesity.
- Reducing alcohol harm.
- Treating drug addiction.
- Reducing smoking rates.
- Improving sexual health.
- Improving mental health.

In Activity 6.2 you are asked to think about how reducing health risks associated with these priorities might help reduce the number of deaths from the two main killers identified earlier.

---

### Activity 6.2         *Critical thinking*

At first glance, some of the above health risks may not seem obviously linked to the two main killer diseases. However, take time to look at each priority in turn and think about how achieving these might also help to reduce deaths from coronary heart disease or stroke and cancer. If you are having trouble thinking of things, try to identify possible physiological changes associated with prioritised health risks, and link these to effects on the heart, circulation or cancer sites. You might then get an idea of how tackling priorities can reduce deaths from the two killer diseases.

*Some possible answers can be found at the end of the chapter.*

---

Activity 6.2 highlights areas of health promotion and illness prevention that nurses can engage in regarding informing, advising and supporting people to get fit and stay healthy. Out-patient, community and practice nurses also give guidance to help people manage a variety of other conditions (e.g. diabetes, asthma) to prevent relapses and reduce hospital readmissions.

## Providing high quality care

While promoting health and preventing ill health have, in recent years, been recognised as key priorities, much of our work as nurses will also be focused on caring for acutely ill patients or those with long-term medical conditions. Government policy in relation to healthcare, in hospital or community settings, prioritises patients' rights to receive a high quality service. Standardised clinical guidelines, as discussed in Chapter 5, are designed to enable a high standard of care to be consistently delivered. In Lord Darzi's NHS review, high quality care was defined as follows:

*High quality care should be as safe and effective as possible, with patients treated with compassion, dignity and respect. As well as clinical quality and safety, quality means care that is personal to each individual.*

(DH, 2008, p7)

In reading this you might be surprised that such fairly straightforward principles should require a high level government-led review. After all, is it not simply saying we should treat people as human beings, care for them, protect them from harm, and help them get better? It is not exactly a 'cutting edge' revelation, is it? The problem is that there have, in recent years, been several well-publicised examples of appalling standards of unsafe, ineffective, uncaring and dehumanising NHS healthcare. Such cases can undermine all the good work that is done, and the public's confidence in the NHS as a whole. Part of the explanation why some hospitals veered away from such basic healthcare values was that they were preoccupied with meeting health targets such as getting more patients assessed and treated more quickly, but they failed to adequately manage the resource implications. This led to overstretched services with staff not coping with demands, and patient care was neglected.

When problems occur in the organisation and delivery of healthcare, the priority is to learn from it and make changes to prevent such things from happening again. In effect, the above definition of high quality care summarises values found in nurses' and other health professionals' ethical codes of practice. Lord Darzi's NHS review team argued that these values need to be applied by everyone working in health and social care, including NHS Trust executives and managers who are responsible for monitoring the quality of care. All healthcare personnel are required to pledge their ongoing commitment to these values, which are enshrined in a proposed new NHS Constitution (see Chapter 10). This represents a contract between healthcare providers and the public, and the future funding of services is dependent on fulfilling agreed terms in delivering high quality care.

Since forming a new government the Conservative/Liberal Democrat coalition has incorporated the recommendations of the NHS review (DH, 2008) in proposals to restructure the NHS so that it is more effective in promoting health, preventing ill health and giving high quality care. In the White Paper *Equity and excellence: liberating the NHS* the coalition endorses Lord Darzi's emphasis on safety, effectiveness and patients' experience in high quality care, as follows:

*The Government's objectives are to reduce mortality and morbidity, increase safety, and improve patient experience and outcomes for all.*

(DH, 2010c, p7)

In order to evaluate healthcare organisations' and professionals' achievements, a new NHS Outcomes Framework is proposed to identify measurable performance indicators, for example, patient-reported outcome measures (PROMs), regarding five key domains (priorities).

*Domain 1:* *Preventing people from dying prematurely.*
*Domain 2:* *Enhancing quality of life for people with long term conditions.*
*Domain 3:* *Helping people recover from episodes of ill health or following injury.*
*Domain 4:* *Ensuring people have a positive experience of care.*
*Domain 5:* *Treating and caring for people in a safe environment and protecting them from avoidable harm.*
(DH, 2010b, p1)

As nurses we have a duty to help to achieve each of these priorities, and Activity 6.3 asks you to think about we might contribute, and how our interventions might be evaluated.

---

**Activity 6.3**                                          *Decision-making*

Look at the five domains of the new NHS Outcomes Framework. For each one, try to identify at least one example of what nurses can do to achieve it and how to measure outcomes of care.

*Some possible answers can be found at the end of the chapter.*

---

Activity 6.3 links the clinical challenges that nurses and other health professionals have to deal with every day (through promoting health, preventing ill health, and in endeavouring to deliver high quality care) to the coalition government's health policy priorities. The main difference between these priorities and the previous government's health targets are that there is greater emphasis on:

- patients' experience and outcomes of care, rather than assuming increasing numbers of people accessing the NHS results in quality care;
- identifying more meaningful patient-centred indicators, such as PROMs, to audit the quality of care;
- assessing, managing and controlling risks to patients' safety in the clinical environment itself, such as preventing cross-infection and injuries;
- integrating health and social care in the community to support those with long-term conditions or disabilities to enjoy a good quality of life.

The priorities in the five domains of the new NHS Outcomes Framework also place more emphasis on NHS Trust executives and managers enabling health professionals to give high quality patient-centred care by ensuring adequate staffing levels, training and equipment. In turn, health professionals are expected to fully consult and collaborate with patients (see Chapter 2), as follows:

*4a) Shared decision-making will become the norm – 'no decision about me without me'.*
(DH, 2010c, p3)

The development and application of PROMs also take patient empowerment a step further than before because the performance of nurses and other health professionals will, in effect, be evaluated by the patients we care for. It underlines the importance of dealing quickly with perceived problems in the organisation or delivery of care so that any harm to patients is prevented, and any inconvenience to them is kept to a minimum.

This is consistent with the requirements of nurses' own professional code of conduct regarding risk assessment and management in protecting the health and safety of patients:

*Manage risk*
*You must act without delay if you believe that you, a colleague or anyone else may be putting someone at risk.*

*You must report your concerns in writing if problems in the environment of care are putting people at risk.*

(NMC, 2008, p6)

The following scenario gives an example of how to manage risk in clinical practice.

---

### Scenario

*Imagine you are on placement in a hospital ward and you are asked to help a more senior student make a bed while the patient has gone to the bathroom. The other student uses the foot pump to elevate the bed so that neither of you has to bend down too far, making the job a bit easier. When the bed is made the senior student thanks you and says she is going for her break but she does not let the bed down for the patient to get back in. What would you do about it?*

1. *Nothing because the other student is senior to you.*
2. *Remind the other student to lower the bed there and then.*
3. *Remind the other student to lower the bed after her break.*
4. *Check again later to see whether the bed was lowered.*
5. *Lower the bed to a safe height yourself without delay.*

---

This scenario, at first glance, may not seem to be a very serious health risk, but there have been a number of fatalities resulting from patients falling out of bed, for example, by the patient banging their head and suffering a brain haemorrhage. Hospital beds are often higher up than beds at home, and floors are usually hard, not thickly carpeted (as they might be at home). Additional risk factors are that patients in hospital may be weaker than normal, and they could be taking medication that makes them drowsy or susceptible to injury. Ensuring that beds are a safe height for patients to get in and out of is, therefore, a health and safety priority.

In the scenario, the patient could come back from the bathroom at any time and try to get back into bed, so if it has not been lowered, the patient will have difficulties, and there is a risk they might fall down. Of the possible responses listed above, 2 and 5 are the only safe options, with 2 being preferable, as the other student might do the same thing again if her memory lapse is not brought to her attention. It is not about 'scoring points' off each other; it is about nurses being committed to ensuring that patients are safe and realising we can all make mistakes, so we need to help each other put these right. The senior student would feel guilty if the patient suffered an injury because she had forgotten to lower the bed.

There are occasions when reminding colleagues of their responsibilities in protecting patients from harm does not work and they continue to put patients at risk, as in the next case study.

## Case study: 'Whistle blowing'

*Between November 2009 and January 2010 the NMC Conduct and Competence Committee reviewed evidence in cases raising concerns about registered nurses' fitness to practise. In one such case, two healthcare assistants gave evidence about the conduct of a registered nurse they worked with at night in a nursing home. They reported that the registered nurse routinely did not follow approved procedures in caring for the residents, which put them at risk. This included: putting double thickness incontinence pads on residents, meaning they could be left soiled for longer; failing to turn residents every two hours to prevent pressure sores despite recording in the nursing notes that they had been turned; and making a habit of sleeping while on duty. The healthcare assistants reported their concerns to the home manager, who investigated and then reported the nurse to the NMC. The NMC judged that the nurse's fitness to practice was impaired, and she was struck off the NMC register.*

The case study is an example of 'whistle blowing' (in which loyalty to colleagues is secondary to protecting the health and safety of those in our care), when inappropriate, unprofessional conduct is reported verbally and in writing to the relevant authorities (e.g. managers, the NMC).

There are also times when nurses and other health professionals 'have their hands tied' in trying to manage risks where there are not sufficient resources to cope with clinical demands. This is where managers and NHS Trust executives bear some responsibility for potentially unsafe working conditions in clinical areas. Organisations such as the Health and Safety Executive (HSE) and Care Quality Commission (CQC) have statutory powers to investigate complaints about unsafe and poor quality provision in hospitals or other health and social care settings. In the earlier scenario we looked at risk management with hospital beds. In a related, real life case, the HSE is in the process of prosecuting an NHS Trust because in November 2007 an 89-year-old male patient fell out of bed and died. The HSE is arguing that the NHS Trust should have ensured bed safety rails were available and fitted to the sides of the patient's bed to prevent him falling, and that by failing to do so they contributed to his death. As nurses we also have a responsibility to inform managers where additional equipment is needed or current equipment needs maintaining or repairing (e.g. suction machine not working). In the next case study the CQC investigate an NHS Trust's management of a mental health unit.

## Case study: Investigation into quality of care

*Between October 2007 and November 2008 six patients died on a ten-bed mental health unit in a community hospital, and this prompted an investigation into the quality of care provided. The findings revealed that there was poor leadership, clinical governance and management of the unit. This included inadequate supervision of doctors, who inappropriately prescribed controlled drugs such as morphine or diamorphine (very powerful painkillers often used in end-of-life care to relieve suffering) to subdue elderly, confused patients suffering from dementia. There were not enough nurses to run the unit safely, staff training was lacking, there was little evidence of effective multi-disciplinary teamwork or decision-making, and record keeping and care planning were also poor. Following discussions with the CQC, the NHS Trust closed the unit in July 2009, as it could not guarantee sufficient staffing levels to provide a safe service.*

In Activity 6.4 you are asked to adopt the role of an investigator in relation to the case study.

---

**Activity 6.4**                                          *Leadership and management*

Imagine you are a member of the CQC investigation team reviewing the quality of care in the mental health unit referred to above. Look at the earlier definition of high quality care from Lord Darzi's NHS review (DH, 2008) and apply it in critiquing the quality of care described in the case study.

*Some possible answers can be found at the end of the chapter.*

---

In Activity 6.4 you were asked to switch perspectives from an 'insider' learning how to be a nurse to an 'outsider' looking in and critically reviewing health professionals' quality of care. In a sense, this is something we need to do continually if we are going to successfully prioritise high quality care for our patients at all times, and it will be further discussed in Chapter 10, which explores **accountability in clinical decision-making**.

This section has explored the influence of health policy in prioritising health promotion, ill health prevention and the provision of high quality patient-centred care. In the next section we look at how nurses use prioritising decision-making skills in dealing with emergency situations.

# Dealing with emergency situations

Effective prioritising in clinical decision-making can mean a patient survives rather than dies from an acute life-threatening episode. As we discussed earlier, preventing people from dying prematurely is a key priority in healthcare, and coronary heart disease or stroke is the biggest cause of deaths in the UK, accounting for over a third of all deaths. As nurses we need to be able to recognise when a patient needs urgent clinical intervention and know what to do about it. In the following case study a student nurse senses something is seriously wrong with a patient.

---

### Case study: Recognising and reporting a medical emergency

*Dennis is at the end of his first year as a student nurse, and he is on a practice placement in a medical ward. One of the patients he has been looking after is Roy, aged 42, who runs a taxi business and was admitted because of a recent history of severe chest pain. Roy has been advised to stop smoking. He has cut down from 20 to 10 a day but finds it too difficult to stop and he regularly goes out for a smoke while on the ward. One day Dennis notices Roy returning from 'his outing' very slowly, looking breathless and pale, clutching his chest, and grimacing. Dennis helps him on to the bed and notices he is sweating profusely. He asks Roy if he is in pain but gets no answer. Dennis tries to feel Roy's radial (wrist) pulse but cannot find it. He informs the ward manager; she takes one look at Roy and tells Dennis to dial the 'crash call' number to alert the duty resuscitation team, and then bring the resuscitation trolley to Roy's bed.*

*continued opposite . . .*

---

*continued . . .*

> When Dennis arrives with the trolley, Roy appears unconscious and the sister is performing cardiopulmonary resuscitation (CPR). She checks that Dennis called the 'crash' team and tells him to elevate the foot of the bed to help blood return to Roy's heart. The 'crash' team arrive (anaesthetist and physician); they help continue CPR, monitor and defibrillate (electrically stimulate) Roy's heart. He is revived, given morphine and transferred to coronary care. The sister tells Dennis he did a good job in recognising something was wrong, alerting her, alerting the 'crash' team, remaining calm, and helping her by doing what she asked without hesitation.

The case study shows that even a first-year student nurse can help prevent the premature death of a patient by: using observation skills (Chapter 3); reporting concerns and collaborating with other team members (Chapter 2); systematically identifying the problem (the absence of a radial pulse (Chapter 4); and following agreed standardised procedures for emergencies (Chapter 5) with guidance from the sister in prioritising Roy's life-threatening episode above all else. The severe pain Roy experienced is associated with myocardial infarction (MI), the death of heart muscle from oxygen deprivation caused by a blood clot or narrowing of the coronary arteries. There is a high mortality (death) rate, as 30 per cent of people experiencing MI for the first time die from it (NICE, 2010b). Survival is improved by immediate diagnosis and intervention, so nurses must recognise a heart attack and administer CPR if there is no carotid (neck) pulse or respiration, which is why the sister began CPR in the case study. In Roy's case, he also needs help to give up smoking as this puts him at risk of further heart attacks by causing blood vessels to constrict. Activity 6.5 invites you to find out more about CPR and the emergency equipment needed.

## Activity 6.5                    *Evidence-based practice and research*

St John's Ambulance advise that all members of the public should learn how to: recognise when someone is having a heart attack; dial 999 or 112 for an ambulance; and do CPR if the patient loses consciousness, stops breathing and there is no pulse. As nurses we should make it a priority to be competent in using these skills, and in checking the contents of the resuscitation trolley. Look this up by searching the literature and checking the up-to-date guidelines provided by the Resuscitation Council (UK) on their website. Practise CPR using a SimMan® or manikin in a skills lab and ask your mentor to quiz you about the resuscitation trolley contents.

*As this is for you to find out about and practise, no specimen answer is provided.*

Activity 6.5 encourages you to develop confidence in being calm and effective when someone needs CPR, a physiological life-saving intervention. In the next section we look at prioritising in the context of psychological interventions to prevent and calm down aggressive behaviour.

# Preventing and de-escalating conflict and aggression

Sometimes prioritising the protection of a patient from harm in clinical settings can involve preventing or de-escalating aggression in them, other patients, visitors or members of staff. Various factors can contribute to patients feeling angry such as: fear about what is wrong with them, previous negative experience, pain, frustration at being kept waiting, feeling not in control of what is going on, separation from friends/family and feeling misunderstood or uncared for. This may escalate as aggressive shouting, verbal abuse, threats or physical abuse towards objects (e.g. slamming doors) or self (e.g. head banging) or other people (e.g. punching). In the following case study a student nurse realises he has provoked a patient to be aggressive.

---

### Case study: Saying sorry to a patient

*When Lawrence was a first-year student nurse (mental health) he was working in a rehabilitation unit. One of the patients, Cecil, aged 57, had a history of a stroke (blood clot in the brain), which resulted in him suffering muscle weakness in his left arm and leg, speech difficulties and a personality change associated with becoming aggressive and violent to others. One day Lawrence was asked by the charge nurse to call the patients to have lunch. Due to Cecil's mobility problems he was slower than the others to respond, and unthinkingly Lawrence said, 'Hurry up, Cecil, it will be cold by the time you get there!' Despite Cecil's disability he lunged at Lawrence, putting his right hand round his throat and squeezing as hard as he could. Lawrence realised he had been insensitive and impatient, looked at Cecil and said, 'I'm sorry, I was out of order.' Cecil released his grip and Lawrence walked with him (at his pace) to the dining room.*

---

The case study shows how Lawrence's initial intervention escalated Cecil's violent behaviour and how his subsequent intervention (saying sorry) de-escalated Cecil's anger and aggression. It also helps to illustrate de-escalation interventions described by Olver (2007).

*   *Active listening* The more we are able to convey that we are interested, attentive and listening to the person's concerns, the better the chances of them ventilating feelings without becoming violent. (Part of Cecil's frustration was due to his speech impairment so there was a greater risk of him expressing anger physically rather than verbally.)
*   *Acknowledging concerns* It helps to confirm that we have understood what the person has said and why they may be feeling frustrated or angry. (Lawrence was suddenly aware that he had been insensitive and impatient and this had understandably angered Cecil.)
*   *Agreeing with truths* When people are angry they are less able to reason and can get more aggressive if we try to argue a point with them. We may want to challenge any unfair comments or abusive language, but the best way we can do this is by not 'rising to the bait', otherwise we are likely to get angry too. Instead, we should try to focus on those parts of a person's tirade that may have a basis in reality regarding perceived injustice. (Lawrence did not try to argue that Cecil's reaction was too aggressive and he did not retaliate with physical force. Instead, he understood he should have been more patient.)

- *Apologising for situation* Where we recognise that a person has a legitimate grievance if we convey we are sorry for what they have had to endure (without taking blame for others) their current level of aggression is more likely to subside. (In the case study, Lawrence *was* at fault, so he apologised for his behaviour, and it worked: Cecil calmed down.)
- *Inviting criticism* Showing that we are prepared to listen to any suggestions to improve services may also reduce a person's possible sense of powerlessness and frustration. As mentioned earlier, enhancing patients' experience and both valuing and responding to their feedback is now a priority in giving quality care (DH, 2010b). (Cecil was not able to articulate his criticism but Lawrence understood his non-verbal criticism very clearly.)

De-escalation techniques are important communication and interpersonal skills used to avoid 'adding fuel to the fire' when people are upset and angry, and all nurses need to develop and practise them. In using them, nurses need to protect themselves by ensuring that other staff are available for support and that they have an escape route should the person become more violent. At this point more specialist mental health nursing skills in managing disturbed behaviour would be required (NICE, 2005), or the police may need to be called to physically restrain the person.

# Supporting long-term carers

Prioritising decision-making in dealing with emergencies or de-escalating aggression is focused on short-term acute episodes in clinical areas that have resources intended to tackle them. As referred to earlier, the quality of long-term care is now also recognised as a priority (DH, 2010b), but this is often provided by a spouse or family member who copes alone, unaware of the support in the community that can help to improve their quality of life and ease the burden of care. In the following case study Pippa, a community nurse specialising in caring for patients with dementia, is asked by the GP to assess a couple as the husband is finding it hard to cope with his wife.

## Case study: Supporting a long-term carer

*Pippa visits Stan, aged 65, and Audrey, aged 60 (diagnosed with Alzheimer's disease, a form of dementia) at their home. She introduces herself but two minutes later Audrey has forgotten who she is. Stan makes everyone a cup of tea and guides Audrey to her favourite chair to sit and listen to music while having her tea. Pippa can see Stan is caring and attentive to Audrey and asks him how long she has needed looking after in this way. Stan explains that Audrey has been like this for five years. She is very forgetful. It is upsetting if they've just got back from somewhere nice and she cannot remember anything about it. She cannot be left alone, as she wanders off and gets lost because she does not know where she is. He gave up work five years ago to take care of her, and he has not had a break in that time. He looks after her 24 hours a day, seven days a week. They have two grown-up daughters who have their own families, do not live nearby, and when they visit Audrey does not recognise them. Stan says they had such great plans for a happy and active retirement travelling the world together, but 'that has all gone out the window now'. Both their savings and pension have been depleted through having to give up work early. Recently he has been feeling guilty for getting angry and shouting at her when she keeps*

*continued overleaf . . .*

continued . . .

> asking the same question over and over again. Stan says he cannot go on like this for much longer, but he does not want Audrey to go into a nursing home.
>
> Pippa discovers Stan has not claimed any disability living allowance for Audrey, and helps him do so, which relieves some of the financial worries. She identifies a mental health day centre that caters for patients such as Audrey, and she now attends three days a week. Pippa also arranges for Audrey to be admitted as an in-patient in a specialist unit for two weeks every year to give Stan a period of respite when he can explore some of the places he wants to visit. Pippa also continues to visit Stan and Audrey. Stan feels his life has been transformed: he does not feel so alone with the responsibility any more. Audrey seems happy at the mental health centre and the unit; Stan can go for walks without worrying about her; and he finds Pippa very understanding.

The case study shows how lay carers do a tremendous job in looking after loved ones, often without having someone to share the burden with, off-duty time, or even an annual holiday. They enable long-term patients to be cared for at home where possible, and reduce their dependence on expensive in-patient or residential health and social care. Supporting carers in the community is vital to enhance the patient's and carer's experience of care and their quality of life together, as demonstrated by Pippa in the case study. An emphasis on patients' experience of care in the NHS Outcomes Framework (DH, 2010b) also supports the application of nurses' caring qualities and skills. Table 6.2 cross-references prioritising in decision-making with nurses' conceptions of nursing in relation to the case study.

| Conceptions of nursing | Prioritising in clinical decision-making |
|---|---|
| Caring | Focusing caring on Stan in recognition of his devotion to his wife and his need for support to help him care for her |
| Listening and being there | Enabling Stan to talk about the problems he faces every day to keep Audrey as safe and well cared for as he can |
| Practical procedures | Implementing changes to improve Stan's quality of life, enabling him to have some time to relax and unwind |
| Knowledge and understanding | Understanding changes to brain in Alzheimer's disease and their effect on cognition, memory, behaviour, mood and personality |
| Communicating | Questioning Stan to assess how he is coping with Audrey, informing him of the range of services that may be of help |

*Table 6.2: Integrating prioritising in clinical decision-making and conceptions of nursing*

| Conceptions of nursing | Prioritising in clinical decision-making |
| --- | --- |
| Patience | Happy to keep reminding Audrey when she forgets her name |
| Teamwork | Liaising with GP, Mental Health Day Centre, in-patient unit to provide alternative care for Audrey and respite for Stan |
| Paperwork and electronic record | Helping Stan complete disability living allowance forms |
| Empathising and non-judgemental | Appreciating Stan's sense of loss at losing the wife he knew yet seeing her every day, and understanding his frustration |
| Professional | Enhancing quality in safety and effectiveness of Audrey's care, her patient experience, and Stan's carer experience |

*Table 6.2: Continued*

## Chapter summary

This chapter explored what is meant when we talk about prioritising in clinical decision-making. Prioritising was closely linked with risk assessment and risk management. Priorities in health policy were then looked at, focusing on health promotion, ill health prevention and giving high quality patient-centred care. Mortality rates were related to policy priorities in reducing the number of premature deaths from main killer diseases such as coronary heart disease. High quality care was defined with reference to the findings of Lord Darzi's NHS review. Case studies of nurses applying prioritising in decision-making to emergency care, de-escalating aggression, and supporting carers of those with long-term conditions were used to link theory to practice.

## Activities: brief outline answers

### Activity 6.1 Reflection (page 89)

Applying risk assessment criteria to, for example, going swimming in a public pool.

a) Predicting/managing uncertainty: will it be crowded? Time visit to avoid school groups.
b) Comparative health risks: good supervision, clearer water, less risky than sea, river or lake.
c) Worst case scenario: bang head or get stuck under water and lose consciousness.
d) Risks to life/health if c) occurs: death from drowning if not rescued by lifeguard.
e) Probability c) might happen: extremely unlikely but fatalities have occurred before.

f)   Maximising safe risk taking: don't dive in shallow end/near water outlet/if pool not clear.

g)   ˙Costs versus benefits of choice: chlorine smell and sore eyes versus very good exercise.

h)   Accountability for decision-making: don't swim if unwell; don't endanger self or others.

## Activity 6.2 Critical thinking (page 91)

You may have included the following points

1.   Tackling obesity: losing weight reduces strain on heart, cholesterol, fatty deposits in arteries (fewer heart attacks): healthy diet five fruit/vegetable daily reduces bowel cancer.

2.   Reducing alcohol harm: cutting down alcohol to safe limits reduces risk of cancer in throat, liver, bowel and breast: also reduces risk of obesity, high blood pressure, stroke.

3.   Treating drug addiction: reduces risk of heart failure or cocaine-induced heart attack.

4.   Reducing smoking rates: reduces risk of cancer of lung, throat and pancreas; also reduces risk of heart attacks, high blood pressure and stroke.

5.   Improving sexual health: safe sex reduces risk of cervical cancer caused by sexually transmitted human papillomavirus; report early symptoms of breast and prostate cancer.

6.   Improving mental health: reducing stress reduces levels of hormones (e.g. cortisone), which in turn reduces risk of high blood pressure, stroke or heart attack.

## Activity 6.3 Reflection (page 93)

Examples of nurses applying NHS Outcomes Framework domains/priorities.

*Domain 1*    *Preventing people from dying prematurely* Ask doctor to prescribe anticoagulant to reduce deep vein thrombosis/pulmonary embolism risk; compare death rates before and after.

*Domain 2*    *Enhancing quality of life for people with long-term conditions* Support patients and carers, co-ordinate community resources, arrange respite care; patients/carers feel supported.

*Domain 3*    *Helping people recover from episodes of ill health or following injury* Help patients address activities of living to aide recuperation, competent interventions; record readmissions.

*Domain 4*    *Ensuring people have a positive experience of care* Keep patients fully informed about available choices and progress, and share decision-making with them; PROMs data.

*Domain 5*    *Treating and caring for people in a safe environment and protecting them from avoidable harm* Use of antiseptic hand scrub between patient contacts to minimise clinical infection rates.

## Activity 6.4 Leadership and management (page 96)

You may have included the following points in your critique of care.

- *Safety of care* Unsafe as an unusually high proportion of the patients died; inadequate staffing levels, teamwork, supervision or management which put patients' health and well-being at risk.

- *Effectiveness of care* Inappropriate prescribing of powerful controlled drugs militated against accurate assessment or therapeutic interventions with elderly patients who were just subdued.

- *Compassion, dignity and respect* Absent due to poor standards of care. Nurses (who could have advocated on patients' behalf) colluded with the treatment regime instead of challenging it.

## Further reading

**Department of Health (DH)** (2010) *Front Line Care: Report by the Prime Minister's Commission on the future of nursing and midwifery in England*. London: DH.

High-level consultation document led by former Prime Minister Gordon Brown involving wide nursing representation and contribution that discussed the implications of Lord Darzi's NHS review and identified priorities for future development of nursing and midwifery services.

## Useful websites

**www.sja.org.uk**

St John's Ambulance website full of useful first-aid information.

**www.hse.gov.uk**

Health and Safety Executive website describing its role and function.

**www.cqc.org.uk**

Care Quality Commission website with links to current and past investigations.

**www.resus.org.uk**

Resuscitation Council (UK) website has up-to-date guidelines on resuscitation.

# Chapter 7
# Experience and intuition in decision-making

---

**NMC Standards for Pre-registration Nursing Education**

This chapter will address the following competencies:

**Domain 3: Nursing practice and decision-making**

5.  All nurses must understand public health principles, priorities and practice in order to recognise and respond to the major causes and social determinants of health, illness and health inequalities. They must use a range of information and data to assess the needs of people, groups, communities and populations, and work to improve health, well-being and experiences of healthcare; secure equal access to health screening, health promotion and healthcare; and promote social inclusion.

---

**NMC Essential Skills Clusters**

This chapter will address the following ESCs:

**Cluster: Care, compassion and communication**

1.  As partners in the care process, people can trust a newly registered graduate nurse to provide collaborative care based on the highest standards, knowledge and competence.
    *By the first progression point:*
    ii.  Works within limitations of the role and recognises own level of competence.

**Cluster: Organisational aspects of care**

10. People can trust the newly registered graduate nurse to deliver nursing interventions and evaluate their effectiveness against the agreed assessment and care plan.
    *By the second progression point:*
    ii.  Works within the limitations of own knowledge and skills to question and provide safe and holistic care.

18. People can trust a newly registered nurse to enhance the safety of service users and identify and actively manage risk and uncertainty in relation to people, the environment, self and others.
    *By entry to the register:*
    xi.  Assesses and implements measures to manage, reduce or remove risk that could be detrimental to people, self and others.

---

## Chapter aims

By the end of this chapter, you should be able to:

- describe how experience and intuition influence decision-making;
- explain the meaning of tacit (embodied/embedded) knowledge and skills;
- relate experience and intuition to examples of clinical decision-making;
- discuss the pros and cons of experience and intuition in decision-making.

# Introduction

Of all the clinical decision-making styles discussed in this book, experience and intuition are the most vague and difficult to describe. Common sense suggests they are an important influence as we tend to be much more effective two months into a practice placement than on our first day, and experienced nurse role models somehow seem to know how to deal with challenging situations.

We are continually adding to our experience as nurses while trying to ensure that patients have a *good experience* of healthcare – this being a health policy priority (Chapter 6) that is reflected in the NMC standards for pre-registration nursing education. To give person-centred care we need to understand and respond to each patient as an individual who experiences things in their own unique way. In order to do this we need to draw on our personal and professional experience and intuition to empathise and communicate with patients, and adapt decision-making and nursing procedures to their particular circumstances.

The following case study links a positive childhood patient experience with becoming a nurse.

## Case study: Childhood memory of being nursed

*Soon after Simon started a pre-registration nursing programme he was asked about his reasons for becoming a nurse. In response, he described an incident he experienced as a young child.*

*'When I was three I was chasing after my brother in the garden when I tripped outside the greenhouse, breaking a pane of glass as I fell, and my arm was bleeding a lot. My mum rushed me to casualty where I had to have an injection and stitches as the wound in my arm was cleaned, sewn up, and bandaged. The nursing staff were so pleasant and polite, especially a male nurse who bandaged up my Teddy bear.'*

The case study suggests that the nurses made a special effort to ensure young Simon had a positive experience of emergency care while also attending to his wound competently. Twenty-two years later the incident was still vivid in Simon's memory, and the nurse he encountered as a child represents an early role model that he now aspires to emulate. Activity 7.1 asks you to reflect on this nurse's decision-making as described in the case study.

The case study reinforces the idea that previous experience influences subsequent decisions, as Simon's childhood experience contributed to his decision to study nursing years later. We do not know how the male nurse developed his understanding of children. It could relate to his own childhood memories, his experience of parenthood or working with children, or the study of developmental psychology. Whatever influenced him, it led to a spontaneous, intuitive decision to bandage the Teddy bear in addition to the standardised wound dressing procedure. This appeared useful in complementing the physical aspects of care with psychological support. We often tap into previous life experience to guide our intuitive judgement and decision-making, but we also need to recognise when we 'are out of our depth' and lack the necessary experience to deliver nursing care competently (see the Essential Skills Clusters at start of this chapter).

This chapter explains what experience and intuition in decision-making means. Research is presented regarding students' development and application of **experience and intuition in clinical decision-making** during their nursing programme and first year as registered nurses. The pros and cons of experience and intuition in nurses' decision-making are then summarised.

# What do experience and intuition in decision-making mean?

## Experience

In general terms experience refers to anything and everything we have ever thought, felt, sensed or done. In addition to predetermined genetic characteristics, the accumulation of life experiences helps to shape our unique individuality and interests, and the choices we make. In this way previous experience motivates us to develop knowledge or skills in particular activities, just as Simon did in relation to the case study. Previous experience can influence how receptive we are to, and how we make sense of the continually changing situations we come across. This is often referred to as 'learning from experience' or as the 'university of life'.

Formal education in schools or universities is a highly regulated learning experience focusing on developing thinking skills that are demonstrated and assessed through written examinations. In contrast, learning from life experience is an informal process focusing on combining practical skills, sensory perception, feelings and thinking skills as appropriate to fulfil particular tasks. In nursing education there is a balance between formal, university-based and informal, work-based learning. This is because nursing is a practice-based discipline that applies a wide range of thinking, emotional, observational, interpersonal and practical skills to patient care. It is not feasible to develop, apply and integrate all these skills without sufficient clinical experience. For example, the male nurse in the case study understood principles of wound healing (thinking skill), noticed how deeply the arm was lacerated by the broken glass (observational skill), empathised with how young Simon was feeling (emotional skill), communicated with him in a friendly and playful way (interpersonal skill), and demonstrated how to bandage a wound (practical skill).

Hence, with experience, we learn, make connections between, and apply thinking, observational, emotional, interpersonal and practical skills to situations. Each person's experience is unique to them, so it is not easy to 'put our finger' on its exact nature; it is only through experience that we can fully integrate theory and practice in delivering holistic (bio–psycho–social–spiritual) care. Activity 7.2 asks you to test this explanation of experience by applying it to your practice.

## Activity 7.2 — *Critical thinking*

As nursing is a practical discipline we can be really sure we have learnt useful skills or knowledge only when we apply them in caring for patients. Identify something you have learned to do as a nurse within clinical practice. Answer the questions below to compare and contrast the skills you applied before and after gaining this practical experience.

1. Describe any nursing activity or procedure you learned to do as a nurse in clinical practice.
2. Use the format below to compare and contrast skills used the first time and the last time you performed the activity:

| Skills used | First time – example of skills | Last time – example of skills |
|---|---|---|
| Thinking | | |
| Observational | | |
| Emotional | | |
| Interpersonal | | |
| Practical | | |

3. Evaluate the effect of experience on your level of competence in using and combining the above skills.

*As this is for you to review your own experience, no outline answer is given, but you may find it useful to discuss your responses and any related development needs with your clinical mentor.*

In completing Activity 7.2 you were asked to do something that may seem slightly unnatural: analysing your experience by relating it to certain criteria (the range of skills). One of the more exciting things about human experience is that it is often spontaneous, unpredictable or even chaotic, and you are never completely sure what is going to happen or how you will react to it. Over-analysing events may therefore seem to miss the point as the true meaning of experience is, arguably, embedded in social contexts and so is only fully understood by participating in them. However, as mentioned before, studying nursing is not restricted to academic lectures; work-based learning in practice is vitally important for us to become competent nurses. We need to develop ways of representing what we do in practice in order to explain or justify decisions and actions, and continually develop a wide range of knowledge and skills. The frequent use of case studies in this book and others in the series helps to portray realistic clinical contexts in which decision-making takes place. Similarly, the activities facilitate learning by asking you to relate the chapter contents to your own clinical experience.

In summary, experience is like an open book of what happens to us throughout our lives, and we are constantly adding new pages to it. The contents of the 'book' are so varied and so extensive it is impossible to be fully conscious of everything we have experienced at any one time. For this reason experience is sometimes referred to as tacit, **embodied knowledge**, meaning it is hidden in our mind somewhere like a forgotten memory. To draw on experience in dealing with similar situations we need to somehow 'index the contents' of our 'book' to aid recognition, recall and application of relevant knowledge and skills lying dormant within us. This is why nurses are required to keep personal and professional portfolios of their clinical experiences (see Chapter 8, Reflective judgement and decision-making). We also need to be attentive to tacit, **embedded knowledge**, which is concealed within the clinical environment or social context we are interacting with. It is as if the social world is a virtual library full of valuable information cues for us to learn from and which can help to trigger memories of things we have observed before and that may be applicable now. Hence, experience informs everyday 'common sense' understanding and decision-making by matching our personal embodied knowledge to information cues embedded in the social contexts we interact with. The following case study helps to illustrate this point.

## Case study: Talking to an unconscious patient

*Nancy and Fred are nursing students on practice placement in a medical ward. They are working together to care for Robert, aged 49, who has been unconscious for more than a week. Robert is able to breathe on his own but is otherwise totally dependent on nurses for personal hygiene, pressure area care, intravenous feeding, catheter care, and gentle flexion and stretching of joints in his arms and legs. Fred asks Nancy, 'Do you think he is ever going to wake up?' Nancy replies, 'There is always a chance that he might.' Sister suddenly appears and gives the pair a solemn look before saying very softly to Robert, 'Your wife called to say she will visit this afternoon.' She again looks Nancy straight in the eye and without saying anything more walks away. The pair both felt that sister was non-verbally 'telling them something' and as the more senior (third-year) student Nancy thought she should know what it was. Then it 'clicked' as Nancy connected in her mind the way sister spoke directly to Robert, the fact that she and Fred were talking about Robert as if he was not there, and being told previously that unconscious patients might still be receptive to sounds (even if they appear unresponsive). She remembered a story about a patient waking up after being in a coma for several weeks during which time his favourite music was played to him, and relatives regularly spoke to him. Nancy follows sister's lead and says, 'Robert, we are going to give you a wash to freshen you up, and Fred will give you a shave so you look smart when your wife comes to see you'.*

The case study demonstrates that nurses can forget things they have experienced or learnt before. When this happens their actions are not evidence-based, and may also be inappropriate. Without 'spelling it out', sister's intervention did enough to challenge Nancy to think more carefully about what she was doing in this particular clinical context. Nancy was then able to piece together the information cues she had missed before and revise her actions. Sometimes connections are formed subconsciously, which is how experience helps to inform intuition.

# Intuition

Intuition refers to a 'sixth sense' or feeling about someone or something or what you should do, without being able to fully explain why or provide any firm evidence to support such 'hunches'. Meeting someone for the first time and making an instant judgement about whether you like or dislike, trust or mistrust, feel safe or unsafe with them involves exercising intuitive judgement.

We are prompted to use intuitive judgement when:

* we have to make up our mind quickly about something;
* we need to attend to many different things at once;
* we do not have scientific evidence to inform decisions.

Intuitive judgement is a subconscious process using pattern recognition to make connections between various information cues embedded in a particular context, weighing up what it all means, and taking appropriate action (Hammond, 1996). Pattern recognition is a holistic way of thinking developed as we attend to various stimuli or cues in adapting to our surroundings. The male nurse in the first case study used intuitive judgement in making use of the Teddy bear (which Simon happened to take along to the hospital with him) to make connections between Simon's young age, physical trauma, anxiety, need for support, and play as a medium of communication.

# Experience and intuition in decision-making

When newly recruited nursing students were asked to describe their understanding of decision-making, many identified experience as a key component. It included significant life events such as marriage and parenthood, and relevant work experience as healthcare assistants (HCAs). In the next case study a student describes being mistaken for a staff nurse when she was an HCA.

## Case study: Mistaken for a staff nurse

*When asked about her decision-making experience Serena said she had worked in a Mental Health Unit for two years as an HCA before starting the nursing programme. No uniforms were worn in the unit, which made it more difficult for newcomers to know who was who at first glance. During her last six months there, Serena said two nursing students allocated to the unit, whom she showed around and explained things to, actually thought she was a staff nurse instead of an HCA. It appeared that Serena's experience had enabled her to learn about and explain the organisation and function of the unit beyond that normally expected of the role. To test out Serena's knowledge and understanding of decision-making further, she was asked to imagine meeting a new patient and then describe how she would go about planning care for this person.*

*continued overleaf . . .*

*continued . . .*

*Serena replied, 'Hopefully I would have some background notes before I went in so I would read those, sit down, have a chat, find out what she needs from me and then I would go about implementing those to the best of my ability. Assess the whole time because things obviously change. I like to write things down so that I can see how I progress and see if I need to change.'*

*Serena's response showed she had learnt to take account of different sources of information for assessment purposes and that patient involvement in care planning is important, demonstrating understanding of how plans can be made responsive to the changing needs of patients. She was also aware of the value of recording information and observations for progress monitoring.*

The case study indicates what can be learnt in clinical practice to aid understanding of care delivery and organisation (without any formal professional education). It does not mean practical experience is a substitute for theory and research, but it emphasises how knowledge and understanding is also embedded in the clinical environment. Effective clinical decision-making integrates theory and practice in matching principles of evidence-based care to the realities and variations of each patient's unique healthcare needs. Hence, as nurses we are intermediaries between explicit, global scientific research and tacit, local experiential knowledge in striving to deliver care that is both evidence-based and patient-centred. This is complex and challenging work. Getting the balance right, where relevant research is applied in a way that takes account of patients' personal needs and preferences, requires practice and experience. Experience also complements the use of collaboration (Chapter 2) and observation in decision-making (Chapter 3) as we develop our repertoire of thinking, practical, observational, emotional and interpersonal skills in interacting with and monitoring the progress of patients we care for.

As we saw in the earlier case study with Nancy and Fred, emulating role models' good practice and learning from our mistakes is also valuable experience that helps enhance decision-making.

As registered nurses after they had completed their nursing programme, the students in Standing's study linked clinical experience with developing and trusting their intuition to deal with challenging **critical incidents** in caring for patients (Standing, 2005). It was as though they had developed 'antennae' that sharpened up their receptivity to what was going on around them, understanding the healthcare implications and guiding how they might respond. This supports an increasing association between practical experience and intuitive decision-making as nurses develop from novice, advanced beginner, competent, proficient, to expert practitioners (Benner, 1984). For the purposes of this book experience and intuition in decision-making is defined as follows:

*Experience and intuition in decision-making is recognising similarities and differences between current and previous situations and being guided by what seemed effective before (and learning from any earlier mistakes) or realising you lack the necessary experience to make a decision.*

# Development of experience and intuition in nurses' clinical decision-making

This section presents research describing the development of a group of nursing students in terms of experience and intuition in decision-making, over a four-year period (Standing, 2005).

## First-year nursing students

Of the 20 students in the research sample, 8 (40 per cent) were aged 17–25 and 12 (60 per cent) were 26–45. Many students therefore had quite a bit of life experience behind them at the start of the nursing programme. All students had previous healthcare experience, and some had a lot.

- Five had less than one year of healthcare experience.
- Eight had between one and five years.
- Two had between five and ten years.
- Five had over ten years of healthcare experience.

Most of the students had worked as HCAs in nursing homes for the elderly, general hospitals, mental health units or a learning disabilities residential care home. Other experience included foster care for autistic children and voluntary work – helping adolescents with epilepsy; answering a student support helpline. One had worked in an ambulance service control centre for ten years, prioritising emergency calls; one dispensed medicines at a pharmacy for 11 years; and one trained as a nurse 20 years before but failed the final exam.

When Simon (the young boy in the first case study of this chapter) was 16 he asked his school for a healthcare placement as a work experience option, mistakenly thinking he would be able to care for people the way he was cared for as a child. Instead, he found himself shaving, washing and toileting elderly men, and this experience discouraged him from studying nursing. However, nine years later (after managing a fast food restaurant) Simon decided he really wanted to be a nurse after all. Other more mature students also felt it was the right time to study nursing now their children were older and less dependent. Parenthood gave them opportunities and experiences in decision-making regarding the care of their children, as the following case study illustrates.

### Case study: Looking after your own child

*When asked to give examples of how she made decisions, Clare described how she used her experience to care for her daughter before seeking medical help.*

*'I had to make an assessment of what was wrong with my daughter. She looked very tired, flushed and unwell, had a sore throat and a bad headache, and complained that the joints in her arms were tender. She lacked energy to do anything, had a high temperature and was 'off' her food. It seemed more than just a cold. I thought it might be flu (influenza) as this can sometimes affect the joints. Either way the GP surgery discourages patients from*

*continued overleaf . . .*

*continued . . .*

*making appointments for such ailments as there is not much they can do, there is a risk of spreading germs, and resting at home is often all that is needed to aid recovery. I gave her 'over the counter' paracetamol and ibuprofen tablets to relieve pain and swelling, and help to lower her temperature, encouraged her to drink lots of fluids and eat what she could, and ensured she had plenty of rest. I got a feeling it was more than flu as she seemed to get a bit better only for same symptoms to recur again. We decided she needed to see a doctor as whatever she had was beyond me. A physical exam and blood test confirmed glandular fever, which is also a viral infection, so there is no cure for it. The recommended treatment was what I was doing already, but at least we knew what was wrong and why it lasted for so long. The GP said it might take a few months for symptoms to go away.'*

The case study is an example of how newly recruited nursing students had relevant previous decision-making experience in caring for others despite lacking professional education. Activity 7.3 asks you to relate the concept of pattern recognition, discussed earlier, to the case study.

## Activity 7.3                                                    *Decision-making*

Earlier it was argued that tacit knowledge and skills (things that are known but are difficult to identify or explain) inform experience and intuition in decision-making. 'Embodied' tacit knowledge is each person's subconscious accumulation of experience, while 'embedded' tacit knowledge refers to information cues in the environment and social context we interact with. We combine embodied and embedded knowledge to make sense of situations we find ourselves in. This involves pattern recognition as we make connections between different information cues.

This activity is intended to help you apply the concept of pattern recognition to the case study.

Clare had no professional healthcare education when she assessed and cared for her daughter so she was not familiar with current evidence-based practice. Instead, she used her experience and intuition to piece together signs and symptoms (information cues), consider alternative causes, make a provisional diagnosis and subsequently question the accuracy of this. Answer the following questions regarding Clare's application of pattern recognition in the case study.

1. Clare thought her daughter's illness was more than a cold and that it could be flu. Why did the pattern of signs and symptoms appear to fit flu rather than a common cold?
2. What did Clare notice in the pattern of signs and symptoms that did not seem to fit flu?
3. What pattern of signs and symptoms is actually shared by cold, flu and glandular fever?

*Some possible answers can be found at the end of the chapter to compare your responses with.*

Collectively, the newly recruited nursing students evidently had a reasonable amount of relevant previous decision-making experience. They referred to five of ten perceptions of decision-making discussed in this book (collaborative, systematic, prioritising, experience, confidence) during their first interview (soon after starting the nursing programme). From this point on, theoretical input and practice placements, associated with the nursing programme, further contributed to their personal understanding, experience and development of clinical decision-making skills.

# Second-year students

By now the students had experienced a range of hospital and community practice placements, which extended their understanding of decision-making. This was highlighted by their reference to the other five perceptions of decision-making discussed in this book (observation, standardised, reflective, ethical sensitivity, accountability). Students associated extra clinical experience and patient contact with a chance to develop their competence in performing practical procedures such as dressings, and understanding how medication and other treatments work. They also appreciated opportunities to gain experience in planning care, as the next case study shows.

## Case study: 'What about this? What about that?'

*Mark recalled how he arranged with his mentor to practise planning care for a patient and how he found being quizzed by the mentor invaluable in getting him to think of things he overlooked.*

*'The first care plan I wrote my mentor said, 'What about this? What about that?' I didn't think of stuff because of my lack of knowledge and experience. The more experience you have of the outcomes of similar cases the more you are able to make a decision about the best pathway.'*

The case study shows how students valued practical experience and mentor support to identify gaps in knowledge and skills, and develop their decision-making competence in planning care.

Students also experienced times when, due to staffing, equipment or organisational problems they felt stressed when mentor support was not available, as the next case study illustrates.

## Case study: Stressful day on the ward

*Hazel described a stressful experience in a surgical ward: 'I went on one day, a staff nurse short, extremely busy ward, four people going to surgery all needed preparation and:*

- *they had to wear a special gown – we hadn't any of those;*
- *they had to have a special bed-pack – we did not have enough of them;*
- *we had to complete forms – the senior student had not done it before and made errors;*
- *we had to take blood pressure (BP) – their electronic BP machines had broken down.*

*I was going to different wards finding this, finding that. The stress was enormous, and at the end of it I went home feeling terrible about the whole thing.'*

The case study illustrates how a shortage of experienced staff and lack of equipment put extra strain on nursing students, trying to compensate for organisational and managerial problems in preparing already anxious patients for major surgery. In effect, it was a lesson in how *not* to deliver high quality care and ensure patients have a positive healthcare experience. It also shows how even inexperienced nursing students in practice placement areas may find themselves in situations where they can make a difference. The next case study further illustrates this.

## Case study: Preventing an accident

*Sally described learning to be alert to unexpected events that she might have to respond to or anticipate and prevent threats to patients' safety if possible during her practice placements.*

*'If I felt it was something I could do, I would get on and do it, especially if that person's life was at risk, or if it was a dangerous situation as they might fall or hurt themselves, or something bad that I could stop from happening. I know I'm only a student and I have to report possible problems to a more experienced nurse, but sometimes if you don't act straightaway, a patient is in trouble. On my last placement the floor was being polished. I noticed that as the cleaner went further up the ward the electric lead got caught on a bed and was suspended above the floor. Maude, aged 77, who was short-sighted and a bit deaf, was walking back to her bed at the time and so I just went up and unplugged the polishing machine to make sure she did not trip over the lead.'*

The case study shows how clinical environments can be hazardous to patients' well-being if nurses and others are not vigilant in continually assessing and controlling health and safety risks. Sally was able to piece together information cues (pattern recognition) in assessing and managing a risk to Maude's safety, realising she might not see the lead and might not hear her warning. Sally's alertness and prompt action may have prevented a fall that could possibly have resulted in a serious injury to Maude. In doing so she was applying activities of living theory to practice in maintaining a safe environment (Roper et al., 2000). Activity 7.4 asks you to think about your experience in contributing to and maintaining a safe environment for patients.

## Activity 7.4                                                          *Reflection*

Identify examples of risks to patients' health and safety in the clinical environment that you have experienced or witnessed and describe information cues that suggested patients were at risk. How can you apply what you have learnt from this experience to maintaining a safe environment for patients in the future?

*As this is for your own reflection, no outline answer is provided.*

# Third-year students

The next time the nursing students were interviewed they were approaching the end of their nursing programme. They were asked to think about how personal, theoretical and practical influences had contributed to their experience in acquiring and applying clinical decision-making skills. Their responses are summarised in the following three case studies.

---

### Case study: Personal influences on experience and intuition in decision-making

*Students identified personal influences as growing up, taking the initiative and second nature.*

a) *Growing up was associated with general life experience outside of nursing programme, which helped students understand patients' or relatives' concerns: 'Life experience has helped a lot. Since starting the course I left home and got married, and we set up our own home. I feel it has helped me to communicate and empathise with patients' partners better than I could before.' Growing up was also associated with personal development that accompanies observing or participating in challenging clinical situations and being responsible for other people's lives as nurses: 'I've grown up. It's definitely a profession where you mature quickly over three years.'*

b) *Taking the initiative was related to a belief that the more you actively participate, the more skills you can develop, and seeking out new learning opportunities in the clinical areas: 'I tend to put myself forward to go and experience things on the ward that other people may not.'*

c) *Second nature referred to learning to trust your experience and intuition in guiding activities that you have developed skills in, and how 'over analysing' can disrupt performance: 'Once you've had the experience you go a certain way without thinking about it too much. It's like if you're walking downstairs and you start thinking about where to place your feet, you fall over.'*
*(Standing, 2005, p100)*

---

The students' ability to identify personal influences in their use of experience and intuition in decision-making supports the idea that becoming a nurse integrates *personal* and professional development. In other words, even academic input has to make sense to students in terms of their own experience otherwise they are unlikely to remember or apply it as they interact with patients. The next case study links theory with experience and intuition in decision-making.

---

### Case study: Theoretical influences on experience and intuition in decision-making

*Just as students felt personal influences (growing up, life experience) benefited professional practice, they also applied theoretical influences (research evidence) to their own personal development needs – 'It was really learning to manage my own time effectively to reduce stress levels, then finding a way to de-stress' – and to their relationships with family, friends and others – 'People know that I've been studying to be a nurse and they approach me and quiz me about their health problems, and they expect me to know what the answers are!'*

*continued overleaf . . .*

*continued . . .*

*The students' integration of theory and research within their experience of nursing practice was mainly related to the earlier discussion of systematic (Chapter 4) and standardised (Chapter 5) decision-making – 'Evidence-based stuff, research, theoretical input about assessment of patients: that, I think, is what most decisions are based on' – and (to be discussed later) reflective (Chapter 8) and ethical sensitivity (Chapter 9) decision-making styles – 'Interpersonal skills, awareness of ourselves, hopefully incorporate into decision-making to avoid making mistakes.'*

*(Standing, 2005, p102)*

Being able to relate theory to our personal experience and understanding is important if we are going to apply it in other situations. Similarly, we need to be receptive to and learn from practice placement experiences and apply this to decision-making, as outlined in the next case study.

## Case study: Practical influences on experience and intuition in decision-making

*The students really valued their practice placements in providing them with so many work-based learning opportunities to develop and apply experience and intuition in decision-making, and to:*

- *interact with patients, relatives, nurses and others: 'You cannot know how much pain someone is experiencing unless you talk to them, so I asked her to describe it to me'; 'Looked at family's ways of communicating with the patient and added it to care plan'; 'Talking with staff about wound assessments, it's all knowledge that is passed on';*
- *emulate experienced role models and mentors: 'Last mentor is a great role model – she looks at the whole picture but also notices very small things that are relevant'; 'I had an excellent mentor who questioned my judgements, helped to draw things out of me';*
- *develop observation skills of patients' well-being: 'Observation is the most important tool; on ward (not hypothetical situations) you base decisions on what you see'; 'Tended to take fluids and supplements in morning, so that was our window of opportunity with patient';*
- *become skilled in performing clinical procedures: 'Gentleman had deep cavity pressure sore, distressed by the smell, dressing had adhered to wound, I needed to use saline to loosen it, I read new dressing should be smaller than wound, so added that to care plan';*
- *assess, plan, deliver, and evaluate nursing care: 'If patient off colour, using your head to work out why'; 'Adapted core care plans, added additional things the patient needed';*
- *reflect and learn from practical experience: 'The way we handled situation wasn't right; vowed next time to do it differently' – 'Supervision groups to reflect, listen and learn'*
- *understand nurses' responsibilities and accountability: 'Been given responsibility, child protection issues to deal with'; 'Lowering the level of observation for a mental health patient is a multidisciplinary decision but if we feel person should go to a higher level of observation that's something nurses do to be safe'.*
*(Standing, 2005, p106)*

The examples given by the students indicate they had developed, integrated and applied their thinking, practical, emotional, observational and interpersonal skills in decision-making. This was associated with more in-depth experience and responsibility in interacting with and caring for patients. A hint of intuitive judgement was suggested, but students' decision-making was mainly guided by procedures, guidelines and experienced role models. Activity 7.5 asks you to relate personal, theoretical and practical influences to your experience.

---

### Activity 7.5            *Reflection*

Identify examples of personal, theoretical, and practical influences in developing your thinking, practical, emotional, observational and interpersonal skills. Describe how you incorporated these skills in developing and applying experience and intuition in your own decision-making.

*As this is for your own reflection, no outline answer is provided.*

---

Activity 7.5 focused on a range of influences in our preparation to become nurses. We now look at what happens once the nursing programme is finished. In the final interview the research sample's experience and intuition in decision-making as registered nurses is described.

## First-year registered nurses

They were registered nurses with 6–12 months' experience when interviewed for the last time. Despite having a preceptorship period to get used to their new role, they found the transition from student to staff nurse very challenging, as the following comments suggest.

- 'Responsibility so great so soon.'
- 'Scary.'
- 'Accountability nightmare.'

Their anxiety was associated with an acute sense of responsibility and accountability, and was compounded by a loss of student status or *'comfort blanket'* and not being able to *'run for help'*.

They also found it a formative period of development, as the following comments show.

- 'Had to learn quickly.'
- 'Thinking on your feet.'
- 'Learnt more since qualifying.'
- 'For that first six months it's a huge learning curve.'
- 'Boundaries for what you feel comfortable doing shift upwards to more complicated things.'

It is as if nothing can fully prepare us for 'coming of age' as registered nurses, and there is no substitute for the experience in being personally responsible and professionally accountable for our clinical judgement, decision-making and interventions in caring for others. Several nurses described examples of developing and applying experience and intuition in decision-making in relation to: 'reading' patients' body language; feeling out of your depth, and assessing patients in emergency situations, as the following case studies illustrate.

> ## Case study: 'Reading' patients' body language
>
> *Serena was a staff nurse in a surgical ward where it was the custom to reposition the beds of patients going for surgery (so they could be observed more closely) when she noticed that a patient looked worried about what was going on.*
>
> *Serena said, 'The lady thought that because we moved her there she was on her way to the morgue because the last patient whose bed was moved had actually died. She never said anything – the fear was in her eyes. I could see she was frightened, so I asked "What's the matter?" I explained, "You were moved because you're a pre-op lady, you can't be too far from the nurses' station as we need to keep an eye on you just to make sure you are alright."'*

The case study illustrates that we need to continually check how patients are experiencing the care we provide and to achieve this we need to be observant, perceptive and responsive to any concerns they may have. It also shows how important it is *not* to assume patients understand what is going on but to take time to explain things to them, preferably before they happen. In the next case study it is the nurse who is anxious and unsure of what is going on.

> ## Case study: Feeling out of your depth
>
> *Simon (from the first case study in this chapter) was now emulating the male nurse who cared for him as a child by working in an emergency care unit. However, when an acutely ill boy was brought in by anxious parents, he felt he lacked the knowledge and skills required to help him.*
>
> *'The little lad was fitting, and it was important he had this drug (Paraldehyde). I felt really bad at having to say, "I'm not happy giving this" because I was unfamiliar with it, and because it was corrosive (it needed a glass syringe as it could eat through plastic). I asked one of the other staff nurses and she said "No" as she had not given it before either. The only person who could give it was the registrar. I felt quite vindicated that I didn't have blame shoved on my shoulders. It was just a lack of knowledge and fear. I'm not a child nurse, but I have to administer drugs to children. You're so paranoid about it you have to check everything. I went home with the drug information and read up on it in my own time so that next time it happens I am happy to give it.'*

Simon knew the boy was acutely ill and needed treatment, and that nurses usually administer medication as prescribed by doctors, but intuitively he felt he was not competent to do it, as shown in Table 7.1.

Experience and intuition is valuable in sensing when we lack the skills to help patients and must avoid harming them through our lack of competence. Experience and intuition in decision-making may also apply subconscious insights that can help patients, as the final case study illustrates.

| Conceptions of nursing | Experience and intuition in decision-making |
| --- | --- |
| Caring | Realising the boy needed specialised skills to care for him |
| Listening and being there | Listening to parents' description of son's fitting episode |
| Practical procedures | Special type of injection procedure requiring glass syringe due to corrosive nature of the drug (Paraldehyde) |
| Knowledge and understanding | Lacked knowledge of drug and no experience in giving it – commitment to learn about it for future reference |
| Communicating | Asked nursing colleague about her experience of drug |
| Patience | Felt vindicated in resisting perceived pressure to give drug |
| Teamwork | Sought out team member team with necessary expertise |
| Paperwork and electronic record | Drug chart; and information sheet about Paraldehyde |
| Empathising and non-judgemental | Understood boy would be anxious to get the right help |
| Professional | Recognised he lacked competence to safely administer injection so declined, to avoid putting the boy at risk |

*Table 7.1: Integrating experience and intuition in decision-making and conceptions of nursing*

## Case study: Assessing patients in emergency situations

*Mark, who had been a staff nurse in an Accident and Emergency unit for nearly a year, explains his understanding of experience and intuition in decision-making in this highly pressurised clinical context.*

*'Someone saying "I've got chest pains" but who looks well and observations are normal is going to wait longer than someone complaining of chest pains, grey, sweaty, pale, short of breath, who just looks awful, and you start processing those things without really thinking about them.*

*In fact, because the nursing station has a clear view where the ambulances pull up, as the doors open we sometimes look at what might be wrong with patients and what triage category (scale of urgency from*

*continued overleaf . . .*

*continued . . .*

*1 immediate resuscitation to 5 non-urgent) we think they're going to be. Once they're in department you talk to them, do a full assessment, and sometimes find we got it right. I think maybe your unease about a patient can come before the exact reasons you're uneasy.*

*I recently saw the guidelines for calling out the medical emergency team, which include things like pulse and respiration, and the last category was 'nurse concern', which they consider equally important. It's a build-up of experience, a kind of unconscious assessment process; you are concerned about a patient but couldn't exactly put your finger on why. That adds to the points score used to decide if a medical emergency team should go to hopefully avert a cardiac arrest.'*

Mark's explanation of experience and intuition in decision-making regarding emergency care reflects many of the points made earlier in the chapter. It involves matching our own personal experience (tacit – embodied knowledge), to what we perceive around us (tacit – embedded knowledge) and using pattern recognition to connect and make sense of information cues. Recognising familiar patterns of signs and symptoms in differentiating one condition and level of urgency from others tends to happen subconsciously and more quickly with experience.

In Activity 7.6 you are asked to think about why clinical settings such as emergency care may prompt the use of intuitive judgement and pattern recognition to guide decision-making.

## Activity 7.6 — *Critical thinking*

As discussed earlier in the chapter, pattern recognition is associated with intuitive judgement and involves making associations between our experience and information cues in our environment. Why do you think emergency care nurses might apply intuitive judgement/pattern recognition?

*Some possible answers can be found at the end of the chapter.*

Activity 7.6 focused on the use of intuitive judgement. Mark's account of experience and intuition in decision-making also showed how it may complement more scientific evidence-based care as we can check out 'hunches' through observations or investigations of various human functions.

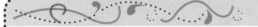

## Chapter summary

This chapter attempted to explain what experience and intuition in decision-making means and how it is developed and applied. We looked at knowledge and understanding hidden in our collection of personal experiences (tacit – embodied), information cues in our environment (tacit – embedded) and how pattern recognition makes connections to inform decision-making. We looked in detail at research following a group of nurses throughout their nursing programme and first year as registered nurses. Case studies demonstrated

*continued opposite . . .*

*continued . . .*

personal, theoretical and practical influences in developing and applying experience and intuition in decision-making. Strengths of experience and intuition included: being receptive to patients' experience of care; attention to holistic range of information cues in clinical contexts; and being able to make quick decisions. Weaknesses included the following: it is a bit vague and 'woolly'; it may be affected by personal biases; and it may be dismissed as unscientific. So where possible it needs to be tested more systematically. In the next chapter we look at more conscious ways of reviewing experiences, learning from them, and applying them to inform reflective judgement in nurses' clinical decision-making.

## Activities: brief outline answers

### Activity 7.1 Reflection (page 106)

You may have included the following points.

1.  Point of bandaging Teddy bear: children learn about the world through play so by bandaging the Teddy bear the male nurse was communicating with Simon at the right level for him to understand about how he needs to protect and take care of his own wound.
2.  Impact of male nurse's intervention: it helped turn a trauma into a positive experience of being understood and cared for by balancing seriousness with the right amount of fun to cheer Simon up and reduce anxiety. The experience contributed to Simon's motivation to become a nurse 22 years later.
3.  Lessons that might apply to adult care: it highlights the need to combine technical and interpersonal skills, communicate at the right level to ensure mutual understanding and collaborate in patient-centred clinical decision-making; and it gives adults a positive experience of healthcare and enhances their future well-being.

### Activity 7.3 Decision-making (page 112)

You may have included the following points:

1.  Flu more severe, more parts of body can be affected including *joints*.
2.  Flu recovery usually within week, recurring symptoms and duration of condition, unlike flu.
3.  All caused by virus, all have cold symptoms (flu or glandular fever have additional symptoms).

### Activity 7.6 Critical thinking (page 120)

You may have included the following points.

*   Intuitive judgement used in A&E as some decisions have to me made very quickly.
*   Pattern recognition used as we need to attend to many things at once, for example, many different patients and having to prioritise who we should attend to first.
*   We may not have scientific evidence we need to inform more accurate decision-making.

## Further reading

**Sharples, K** (2011) *Learning to Learn in Nursing Practice*. Exeter: Learning Matters.

Useful chapter on learning from experience in practice setting where decision-making takes place.

# Chapter 8
# Reflective judgement and decision-making

*continued opposite . . .*

*continued . . .*

> *By entry to the register:*
> xii. Assesses, evaluates and interprets risk indicators and balances risks against benefits, taking account of the level of risk that people are prepared to take.

## Chapter aims

By the end of this chapter, you should be able to:

* explain how reflection converts experience into learning;
* give examples of reflective judgement and decision-making;
* distinguish between reflective and intuitive decision-making;
* apply reflection in personal and professional development;
* understand what reflexivity means and be able to apply it;
* identify the pros and cons of reflective decision-making.

# Introduction

This chapter looks at reflective judgement and decision-making in clinical practice. As nurses we are expected to reflect on our experiences to learn how to improve care we give to patients (professional development) and learn about ourselves in the process (personal development). It is evident in the NMC *Standards for pre-registration nursing education* (NMC, 2010a), which emphasise self-awareness and reflection to convert experience into learning. It is also reinforced by the requirement to keep up-to-date professional portfolios in order to log observations, activities and reflections in our ongoing development as nurses. These portfolios are important because they form part of nursing students' assessment, and following registration as nurses, they give potential employers an indication of whether our skills match job requirements.

Recording experiences and reflections is also a useful way of researching how nurses develop and apply clinical judgement and decision-making skills. Each type of decision-making identified in this book came from students reflecting on their development in becoming registered nurses (Standing, 2005). Like experience and intuition (Chapter 7), reflective decision-making is based on clinical experience. The main difference between intuitive and reflective decision-making is that the former is subconscious and spontaneous while the latter is conscious and deliberate. The following case study helps to illustrate some differences between these two styles.

## Case study: Why did I say that?

*Second-year nursing students were asked to reflect on their practice placement experiences. They described a range of 'critical incidents' they had been involved in, been affected by and learnt from. Many of these occurred while interacting with patients or relatives where students were less closely supervised than when performing specific clinical procedures. They were, therefore, more self-reliant at these times, judging what to say or not say, according to their appraisal of the situation and any relevant experience. Heather, a mature nursing student in a surgical unit, was very self-critical when describing how she had responded to a patient.*

*'A lady waiting to go to surgery said, "My husband died six months ago and it's times like this I really wish he was here and I could say go and get us a cup tea, love." I didn't think and said, "Oh yes, well thank goodness I have got my husband at home because he would be running around after me." As soon as I said it I thought, "You stupid woman! Why did I say that? She must have thought what an insensitive thing for me to say" [At this point the interviewer asked Heather to think of an alternative way of responding] I should have just said, "You must really miss him and for safety reasons we cannot give you a drink before surgery, but when you come back from theatre, and you have recovered from the anaesthetic, we'll make sure you get a cup of tea."'*

*We don't actually know if the lady was upset by Heather's response. Heather was self-critical for answering without thinking, which led her to talk about herself rather than being focused and sensitive to the patient's feelings. She realised her misjudgement straightaway but the moment had passed and she did not feel able to make amends at the time. Heather's disappointment prompted further reflection, resulting in her identifying a more appropriate response. From this incident she learned to think more carefully about what she said to patients, to be wary about the appropriateness of self-disclosure, and to value communication skills as nursing interventions.*

The case study highlights differences between intuitive and reflective decision-making. Heather intuitively and spontaneously disclosed information about her husband and then with hindsight reflected, reviewed what happened, and learned to respond in a more patient-centred manner. Because intuition is a subconscious process it is difficult to analyse, so we can only really judge if it is accurate when reviewing outcomes of intuitive decisions. We have no reason to question our intuition if we seem to be getting on well with other people. However, when Heather became aware that she was talking about her own husband, she put herself 'in the lady's shoes' and realised it was an insensitive and unhelpful thing for her to say. Through reflection she learnt to balance rapport, sensitivity to patients and achieving therapeutic goals (e.g. being supportive while indicating it was not a good idea to drink tea before having surgery). Activity 8.1 invites you to use reflection in reviewing an interaction you have had with a patient.

## Activity 8.1         *Reflection*

As mentioned above, when we converse with others we tend to draw on our own experiences and sometimes we may not even realise we are doing it. As nurses it is important to develop a good rapport with patients, but it can be tricky to strike the right balance between

*continued opposite . . .*

*continued . . .*

being friendly and being professional in the way we communicate. Think about the conversations you have had with patients and see if you can recall times when you did not know what to say, or you felt you said the wrong thing, or the patient or relative appeared upset with what you were saying. Then answer the following questions in order to complete your own reflective cycle.

• Describe an incident in as much detail as you can (what happened, when, where, who with).
• Write down how this made you feel and how you think the patient or anyone else involved may have felt (e.g. were you self-critical like Heather was?).
• Identify why you felt the way you did (e.g. Heather was angry with herself because she thought she was 'a stupid woman') and whether you have had similar thoughts or feelings before.
• Describe what, with hindsight, you might have done differently to achieve a better out-come.
• Explain how you might apply lessons from this reflective exercise in your future inter-actions.
• Test it out next time you find yourself in a similar situation and note whether you feel more self-aware in how you communicate with patients, and if this helps you address their needs.
• Reflect on what you have learned about balancing skills in establishing rapport, sensi-tivity to patients and achieving nursing goals. Write up this exercise in your professional portfolio.

*As this activity is for your own reflection, no specimen answer is provided.*

Both the case study and Activity 8.1 reinforce the idea that reflection is valuable in facilitating professional and personal development by converting experience into learning. This can then be applied to inform future clinical judgement, decision-making and nursing interventions. It is often prompted by an awareness that something did not go as well as it should have, and this may result in self-denigration (like Heather) or in blaming others. To avoid getting stuck in such negative emotions we need to use these incidents as learning opportunities, work out how we can improve, test it out, review progress and continually develop ourselves as nurses and as people.

This chapter: clarifies what reflective judgement and decision-making in nursing is; explores ways that reflection can convert experience into useful learning; looks at how reflective decision-making involves integrating personal, theoretical and practice knowledge, and associated skills; explains the importance of **reflexivity** in reflective clinical decision-making; and, finally, summarises the pros and cons of reflective judgement and decision-making in nursing.

# Reflective judgement and decision making in nursing

When nursing students were asked about their perceptions of clinical decision-making they described how reflecting on practical experience and interactions with patients helped them to understand and develop their role in contributing to nursing decisions and actions:

> *It is important to be internally reflective. If you don't think about your experiences you don't learn from them, how it has affected you and other people, and what you would do differently next time.*
> (Standing, 2005, p89)

The students found this form of experiential work-based learning very different from the academic input, theory and research they studied at university. In practice placements what they needed to learn was not made explicit in a PowerPoint presentation; it was embedded in the clinical context itself in recognising and addressing patients' constantly changing healthcare needs. One student described how this put more responsibility on her to make sense of things:

> *You have to put things together in your mind and make connections because the books don't always. You have to be able to work things out for yourself.*
> (Standing, 2005, p88)

Like experience and intuition (Chapter 7) reflective decision-making involves nurses relating personal experience (embodied knowledge) to information cues in clinical practice (embedded knowledge). Getting to know patients enables us to recognise changes in patterns of behaviour, speech or facial expression and the possible healthcare implications, such as recognising when an asthmatic person urgently needs to inhale a drug to dilate their air passages. Through reflection this 'taken for granted' tacit (hidden) embodied and embedded knowledge and skills can be identified, made more explicit by describing it, and perhaps related to relevant theoretical principles. Table 8.1 summarises the similarities and differences between intuitive and reflective decision-making.

Table 8.1 also illustrates how reflective decision-making involves consciously reviewing experience and taking time to deliberate about what the best course of action is. The delay in decision-making can be relatively short – such as taking a minute to think of what to say when you notice a visitor has given a newly diagnosed diabetic patient a large box of milk chocolates – or it can take much longer – such as judging whether a patient who has been treated for depression after attempting suicide is now well enough to be discharged from an acute mental health unit. Thinking about what action to take when interacting with patients is called reflection-in-action and taking time out to look back at what happened and learn from it is called reflection-on-action (Schön, 1983). In the case study earlier in this chapter Heather was aware she had made a mistake when talking to the lady waiting to go to surgery but she was unable to think of an alternative intervention at that time. Looking back at the incident she was able to think of a better response through her reflection-on-action.

The practice-based nature of reflective decision-making therefore complements experience and intuition (Chapter 7), observation (Chapter 3), and collaborative decision-making (Chapter 2) for

| Focus of comparison | Intuitive decision making | Reflective decision making |
|---|---|---|
| Main source of information | Practical experience | Practical experience |
| How information processed | Pattern recognition | Pattern recognition |
| Use of nursing knowledge | Tacit (embodied, embedded) | Make tacit knowledge explicit |
| Level of mental awareness | Subconscious | Conscious |
| Speed of decision-making | Immediate | Delayed |
| Type of decision-making | Spontaneous | Deliberate |
| Explaining decision-making | Felt it was right at the time | Describe personal rationale |
| Auditing quality of decisions | Patient outcomes | Rationale and patient outcomes |

*Table 8.1: Comparing and contrasting intuitive versus reflective decision-making*

nursing care to be patient-centred and relevant to their needs and preferences. The ability to explain one's reasons for decisions and how they are intended to benefit patients also means that the process of reflective decision-making is auditable. This is important for professional accountability as nurses *must deliver care based on the best available evidence or best practice* (NMC, 2008, p7). While evidence-based practice is usually associated with applying research through systematic (Chapter 4) and standardised (Chapter 5) decision-making, nurses' observations and reflections can often provide valuable evidence to support best practice. This is strengthened where nurses can demonstrate working through different steps of a reflective cycle, just as you did when reflecting on your interaction with a patient in Activity 8.1. For the purposes of this book, reflective decision-making is understood to mean the following:

> *Reflective decision-making is a conscious and deliberate process informed by learning from previous experience and it has a 'personal rationale' that can be explained to others. It involves pausing for thought to review events as they occur (reflection-in-action) and choose the best nursing option or to review past events (reflection-on-action) and help to inform future practice.*

# Using reflection to convert experience into useful learning

We can use reflection to review and learn from our experiences individually, with someone else, or in group situations. In the following case study Jo, a second-year nursing student describes her own private way of disentangling what has happened in the clinical area in order to 'unwind' and relax when she goes home.

---

### Case study; Thinking things through in the shower

*'When I get home from a shift I would be straight in the shower and think about things: Why did I do that? What led to it? Should it have happened? If I was there again, having hindsight, would I do it that way?*

*I think it through in the shower, which is my thinking space, and when I come out I leave it behind because if we kept everything with us continually and thought about it 24 hours a day we would all go loopy, but I could spend 45 minutes in the shower contemplating things.'*

---

The case study suggests that a lot can happen during a shift and there may not be time to 'take it all in', which poses questions or 'food for thought' for when there is more time to reflect on events. Jo found working through her own reflective cycle, to make sense of her experience in clinical practice, necessary and beneficial in order to disengage from work ('leave it behind') when she got out of the shower. If she did not create space for reflection, Jo suggests she would remain stressed ('go loopy') as things might continue to nag her. Jo uses the ritual of showering (washing the cares of the day away) in a very positive way to aid her reflection. Hence, there may be occupational health benefits for nurses and other health professionals to have opportunities for reflection. It also contributes to lifelong learning and professional development, as indicated by Jo in casting a critical eye on what she might do to improve her effectiveness as a nurse. Activity 8.2 asks you to critically review the value of individual reflection as described by Jo.

---

### Activity 8.2                                        *Critical thinking*

Do you, like Jo, have your own individual way of reflecting back on what has happened in clinical practice? What do you think are the strengths and weaknesses of using individual reflection to convert experience into useful learning?

*Some possible answers can be found at the end of the chapter.*

---

Sometimes it may be easier to reflect on incidents when discussing them with someone else, such as a friend, colleague or mentor. In the first case study Heather was still 'stuck' at being angry with herself until she was asked to think of an alternative response, which helped her to 'move on'. In Chapter 4 nursing students acknowledged how being questioned by their mentors helped them to identify things they had not thought of before when planning systematic care. Supportive and challenging mentoring and supervision in nursing can, therefore, facilitate the development of clinical competence in reflective decision-making (Standing, 1999). Activity 8.3 asks you to think about how you might discuss your reflections with someone else.

Have you shared your thoughts and feelings in reflecting on clinical experience with another person? What 'ground rules' do think are important to adhere to for this to be effective? How might reflecting with someone else be more or less effective than reflecting on your own?

*Some possible answers can be found at the end of the chapter.*

As we saw in Chapter 2, many clinical decisions are collaborative, involving contributions from different healthcare professionals, as described by one of the students:

> *Decisions on the ward are normally part of a multidisciplinary thing, rather than just one individual saying, 'This is how it's going to be', because others will bring different insights to the situation. So, by having more of you, you can get a better approach.*
> (Standing, 2005, p86)

It seems sensible, then, to have opportunities for team members to reflect on events together, as needed. In the following case study Clare, a second-year nursing student in a children's unit, recalls her first experience of group reflection and the benefits she associated with it.

### Case study: Talking it through

*'We had a terrible day on my placement: a baby died first thing; we had a horrendous non-accidental injury; and then a GP sent in a child with leukaemia. The nice part was at the end of the shift everyone sat down and talked about it. The doctors were there as well. I had never seen that before and although I didn't have much input I didn't feel the need because I was listening to what the team had to say. The importance of reflection was really brought home to me that day. It did actually prompt me to look more at the child protection issue.'*

*(Standing, 2005, p86)*

Any one of these events is challenging to deal with, but all three occurring together during the same shift must have been extremely demanding both emotionally and professionally. The death of a baby is a tragic loss for the parents, and can affect nurses and other team members, too, while they are also trying to be sensitive to the parents' grief. A non-accidental injury is disturbing because it is usually caused by adults entrusted to care for the child, and the healthcare team have a legal responsibility under the Children Act 1989 to report it immediately to social services, to ensure the child is protected from further abuse. On top of this the team needed to care for a newly admitted seriously ill child who was suffering from leukaemia (cancer of the white blood cells).

Despite feeling 'out of her depth' Clare was positive about it because she had participated in an inter-professional support group, which was a unique and productive experience for her. The team appeared to recognise that too much had happened for nurses, doctors and others to leave the unit without reflecting on the events in a supportive atmosphere. This type of reflection was not just checking whether the right decisions and actions had been taken; it also enabled staff to express their feelings about the traumatic events in a non-judgemental manner. Being sensitive to each others' need to de-stress can help health professionals be more sensitive to patients because they feel less overwhelmed by their own emotional baggage. Acknowledging and ventilating emotions (catharsis) can also help to 'clear the mind', enabling nurses and others to develop deeper understanding and focus on what they need to do (Heron, 1989). Witnessing the above events and listening to her colleagues helped Clare to value reflection. This prompted her to fill a gap in her own knowledge regarding child protection policy and procedures, and nurses' responsibilities in applying them. In Activity 8.4 you are asked to think about participating and reflecting on your practice in an inter-professional support group.

---

### Activity 8.4                  *Team working*

Have you had any experience in contributing to healthcare team discussions or participating in supportive, therapeutic or supervisory group work? How might group reflection by a healthcare team remove or reinforce barriers to effective inter-professional teamwork and decision-making?

*Some possible answers can be found at the end of the chapter.*

---

This concludes our look at the different ways of converting experience into useful learning by reflecting on practice individually, in pairs or in groups. In the next section we look at the range of knowledge and skills that are developed, integrated and applied in reflective decision-making.

# Integrating personal, theoretical and practical influences

Becoming a nurse involves both personal and professional (theoretical and practical) development. As a nursing student you begin the programme with a unique personal history and outlook, and all the theory, research and work-based learning you experience is filtered through and interpreted by your own values and expectations. The further you progress through the programme the more opportunities there are to integrate increasing amounts of theoretical and practical knowledge in your personal experience of becoming a nurse. Reflection is a means to connect and integrate personal, theoretical and practical worlds. In the next case study Mark, a second-year student, reflects on his professional development.

## Case study: Satisfying to teach a procedure

*'The new experience of being a student on the wards was quite difficult to enjoy at first because you felt incredibly useless, so when people were busy there was very little I could do. I enjoy my placements much more now that I have got more competent in certain practical skills. I've come to value the clinical skills that I have been learning more than perhaps I did at the start. I was focusing more on the person-to-person aspect then. I get self-esteem from being caring, someone the patients get on with, but also from being able to do technical things that perhaps they don't understand. I have found it very satisfying to teach a procedure to a student nurse (who was earlier on in the programme than me), that I had a skill they didn't have that I could impart to them.'*

Like many nurses, Mark appears to get personal satisfaction from being useful in helping to care for patients. This ambition was initially frustrated by his lack of knowledge and skills, but then he developed competence in practical skills to a level that he could teach more junior students. The technical nature of some skills also required a theoretical understanding to fully appreciate their use and purpose. Figure 8.1 summarises how personal, theoretical and practical influences are integrated in an ongoing experiential learning cycle (adapted from Kolb, 1984) where reflection has a key role in making sense of experience, and shaping future decisions and interventions.

*Figure 8.1: Reflective decision-making: a personal / practical / theoretical / experiential cycle*

In Figure 8.1 the most important stage of the cycle is practising nursing care, but in order to ensure that this is well informed and continually adjusted to be relevant in addressing patients' changing circumstances, the other stages of the cycle are also needed. The various decision-making styles discussed in this book complement some stages of the cycle more than others, for example: practising nursing care – experience and intuition; reflecting on practice – reflective; theorising about nursing – ethical sensitivity; planning patient care – systematic; and personal interpretation – confidence. Ultimately, nurses' judgement and decision-making are personal choices that we are professionally accountable for. This is why personal interpretation lies at the heart of this adapted experiential cycle both influencing and influenced by each of the stages.

The experiential model of reflective decision-making is strongly grounded in and matched to holistic patient-centred care and clinical contexts in which it is delivered. It requires nurses to apply a range of thinking, practical, emotional, interpersonal and observational skills, including, but not limited to theory and scientific research where relevant to patient care. This holistic view of reflective decision-making is supported by multiple intelligences theory (Gardner, 1983), which identifies linguistic, logical-mathematical, spatial-visual, bodily-kinaesthetic, musical-auditory, interpersonal and intrapersonal forms of intelligence complementing the above range of skills. Logical-mathematical intelligence is the most analytical form, which is usually associated with scientific and theoretical concepts. As such, it links with 'Theorising about nursing' in Figure 8.1 and supports critical thinking associated with reflexivity in decision-making, as discussed next.

# Reflexivity in reflective decision-making

This chapter has made a case for the importance of reflective decision-making in nursing, but it can be open to criticism for potential personal bias or misinterpreting information cues. There may be a greater danger of this where nurses are reflecting individually rather than in pairs or groups. It is not always possible to test out our interpretation of events or proposed actions with others and, in any event, we are individually accountable for our decisions. It is therefore wise to find a way of self-monitoring our judgement and decision-making for possible inaccuracies. This means assuming that our interpretations could be wrong, finding ways to test them, and being open about our potential biases. Researchers call it reflexivity, which basically means critically examining the way we reflect on our experience and interpret observations. When applied to clinical decision-making, reflexivity has been defined as follows:

> *Lifelong learning in the critical self-examination of ideas, assumptions, biases and any lack of knowledge or understanding that may impede sound patient-centred clinical judgement and decision-making, plus a commitment to take action and improve knowledge and skills.*
> (Standing and Standing, 2010, p214)

Applying reflexivity in reflective decision-making is particularly important to accurately assess serious health risks. We will look at two case studies using critical incidents (events having a significant impact, prompting us to reflect and learn from them) with contrasting outcomes.

## Case study: I was angry with myself

*Mark has been a staff nurse in an Accident and Emergency unit for nearly a year. One day Derek, 35 years old, is admitted because he has become confused. He is accompanied by his wife. Mark assesses Derek, not knowing he was in a car accident 24 hours before and sustained a head injury. Derek is too confused to mention it and his wife does not either because he had a skull X-ray in another hospital and they didn't find anything wrong. Derek has suffered a brain haemorrhage and dies within a couple of hours. Mark blames himself for not considering the possibility that Derek's symptoms were caused by a head injury.*

*'I was very angry with myself. I'd made an assumption and continued down that route until it was forcibly thrust to my attention something was very wrong. When I'm working in A&E I can get influenced by paramedics' assumptions, and that's 'tripped me up' a couple of times. If a paramedic has a preconception that a patient is faking it, I have to work very hard not to think the same. It's not the nursing role to make a medical*

*continued opposite . . .*

*continued . . .*

*diagnosis but we have to pick an appropriate category to do the triage (prioritise most urgent cases). From that incident I learnt to be:*

- *less fixed in what I think;*
- *less dependent on what other people think;*
- *more ready to make my own decisions.*

*Initially I learnt the wrong lessons. The next day another patient was unwell, we didn't know why. He was in the same cubicle and was my responsibility. I was very anxious and wanted a doctor to see him immediately. The doctor had a quick look and said he'd be alright, probably just had a transient ischaemic attack (temporary lack of oxygen to the brain) – the same provisional diagnosis I had incorrectly attributed to Derek. I was getting upset. I had to take off and say to myself, "Calm down, it's not the same patient, it just feels the same", because I felt sure if I didn't get help immediately he was going to die as well.'*

The case study highlights the life-and-death nature of many nursing decisions, the fine line between these possible outcomes, and how making errors can shake confidence. In doing so it conveys some limitations of reflective decision-making in that it depends on the quality of available information such as identifying an accurate history of the onset of a patient's illness and current symptoms. Unreliable witnesses who withhold relevant information or make inaccurate assumptions can cloud your judgement. Relying upon observation and reflection to the exclusion of more scientific evidence may result in relevant research being ignored. From this incident Mark learned to be reflexive in evaluating opinions and advice he received (*less dependent on what other people think*) to think for himself (*make my own decisions*) and acknowledge the tentative nature of his decisions (*learnt to be less fixed in what I think*). In Activity 8.5 you are asked to explore the concept of reflexivity in more depth.

## Activity 8.5        *Evidence-based practice and research*

Do an online literature search on the concept of reflexivity, including qualitative research in which it is often applied to demonstrate control of researcher bias. Devise your own working definition of reflexivity that you can apply in critiquing the accuracy of your reflective decision-making. With reference to your definition, develop a couple of questions that can test your reflexivity.

*As this is for your own personal research, no specimen answer is provided.*

In the previous case study Mark's reflexivity swung from being underdeveloped when he was unaware of the seriousness of Derek's condition to being overdeveloped after Derek died, when he no longer trusted his powers of observation and reflection. The change was influenced by Mark's emotional distress in failing to detect the head injury and being unable to save Derek's life. This illustrates how stressful registered nurses' decision-making responsibilities can be. It reinforces the point made earlier about the need to talk about traumatic events in a supportive setting, and highlights the need for reflexivity to reduce bias and inaccuracy in decision-making.

In the next case study Clare, a staff nurse in a children's unit, is faced with an emergency she does not feel experienced enough to deal with but has to as she is the only nurse present.

## Case study: He's not breathing

*Clare recalled a mother approaching her suddenly, in a state of distress.*

*'The lady shouted, "He's blue, he's not breathing!" and threw this baby into my arms. There wasn't anyone with me, no one in shouting distance. I was shocked by the urgency of a situation I was not prepared for, but something in the back of my mind helped me to assess, realise this child had an obstruction in his airway, and realise that I needed to clear it immediately. I laid him face down on my lap and patted his back four times, he coughed, some thick mucous came up, and he started breathing again and changed back to his natural colour. If I hadn't been taught what to look for, I wouldn't have been able to do it. I just pictured [Nurse Tutor] explaining what to look for in a child with severe respiratory distress and what to do. Afterwards we had a reflective talk on the unit and it was nice to know I had done everything the senior member of staff would have done.'*

The critical nature of the baby's condition and the absence of immediate support meant that Clare found she was alone with the responsibility of reviving the baby, with a very anxious mother in attendance. She managed to remain sufficiently composed in these challenging circumstances, and in the absence of relevant previous practical experience, dealt with the emergency. Clare's ability to understand what was wrong and what she needed to do about it involved 'reflection-in-action', matching her observations of the baby to recollection of a lecture and video at university regarding identifying and relieving an obstructed airway in a baby. Clare did not actually feel competent to deal with the emergency; if a more experienced person had been present, she would have deferred to them. But the baby was blue and had stopped breathing. If she went looking for someone else to help it might be too late to save him, so although she had not done it before she felt she had to try to revive the baby. Table 8.2 shows how Clare integrated reflective decision-making with conceptions of nursing.

| Conceptions of nursing | Reflective clinical decision-making |
|---|---|
| Caring | Doing everything possible to help the baby breathe |
| Listening and being there | Being attentive and responsive to mother's cry for help |
| Practical procedures | Using an approved method to unblock the airway |

*Table 8.2: Integrating reflective clinical decision-making and conceptions of nursing*

| Conceptions of nursing | Reflective clinical decision-making |
|---|---|
| Knowledge and understanding | Linking baby's appearance with respiratory distress |
| Communicating | Trying not to show how worried she was |
| Patience | Not panicking when confronted by the emergency |
| Teamwork | Reflecting and receiving supportive supervision after incident |
| Paperwork and electronic record | Recording what happened in the nursing records |
| Empathising and non-judgemental | Understanding how distressing it was for mother and baby |
| Professional | Carrying out effective risk assessment and management of emergency |

*Table 8.2: Continued*

## Chapter summary

This chapter presented different aspects of reflective decision-making in nursing, which were related to personal and professional development in converting clinical experience into useful learning through reflection-in-action and reflection-on-action, privately, in pairs or in groups. The patient and practice-centred basis of reflective decision-making was compared and contrasted with experience and intuition in decision-making. It was argued that reflection helps to articulate personal and practical knowledge that remains hidden in intuitive decision-making. An experiential reflective decision-making model was proposed, integrating personal, theoretical and practical influences and associated thinking, practical, emotional, interpersonal and observational skills. This closely complements the principles of holistic nursing care. Examples and case studies of reflective decision-making in different pathways from junior nursing student to registered nurse were provided, together with a variety of activities to help readers relate theory to practice. The strengths of reflective decision-making include: its relevance to patient-centred care; its recognition of the importance of information cues and observations in the clinical context; and its contribution to 'grass roots' nursing knowledge and expertise. The weaknesses include: its local focus, which might mean it ignores relevant national research that could benefit patients; the fact that it is limited by the quality of observations and available information cues; and the potential for bias and inaccuracy by decision makers when interpreting experience. It was argued that the concept of reflexivity, borrowed from qualitative research, is valuable to raise awareness and control of personal bias by testing out assumptions where possible.

## Activities: brief outline answers

### Activity 8.2 Critical thinking (page 128)

You may have included the following points.

Strengths
- Time and place of one's choosing.
- As often as you like.
- Privacy and peace.
- Autonomy – self-care.

Weaknesses
- Limited perspective.
- Support not available.
- Views unchallenged.

### Activity 8.3 Communication (page 129)

You may have included the following points.

Ground rules
- Agree aims.
- Clarify roles.
- Confidentiality clause.

Pair more or less effective than individual
- Dependent on both adhering to agreed ground rules.
- Less effective if collusion occurs.
- More effective if trusting, honest, supportive and challenging.

### Activity 8.4 Team working (page 130)

You may have included the following points.

Reduce barriers
- Group perceived to be relevant by team members.
- Opportunities for interaction and mutual understanding.
- Possibly enhance effectiveness of integrated care pathways.
- Identifying, valuing and pursuing shared objectives.

Reinforce barriers
- No consensus about perceived need for group.
- Group members do not have equal status.
- Used to criticise or embarrass colleagues.
- No values or objectives shared by group.

## Further reading

**Howatson-Jones, L** (2010) *Reflective Practice in Nursing.* Exeter: Learning Matters.

Many interesting case studies of learning through reflection particularly relevant to adult nursing.

# Chapter 9
# Ethical sensitivity in decision-making

## NMC Standards for Pre-registration Nursing Education

This chapter will address the following competencies:

### Domain 1: Professional values

4. All nurses must work in partnership with service users, carers, families, groups, communities and organisations. They must manage risk, and promote health and well-being while aiming to empower choices that promote self-care and safety.

## NMC Essential Skills Clusters

This chapter will address the following ESCs:

### Cluster: Care, compassion and communication

2. People can trust the newly registered graduate nurse to engage in person-centred care empowering people to make choices about how their needs are met when they are unable to meet them for themselves.

    *By the second progression point:*

    ii. Actively empowers people to be involved in the assessment and care planning process.

4. People can trust a newly qualified graduate nurse to engage with them and their family or carers within their cultural environments in an acceptant and anti-discriminatory manner free from harassment and exploitation.

    *By the first progression point:*

    iii. Adopts a principled approach to care underpinned by the Code (NMC, 2008).

    *By entry to the register:*

    v. Is acceptant of differing cultural traditions, beliefs, UK legal frameworks and professional ethics when planning care with people and their families and carers.

8. People can trust the newly registered graduate nurse to gain their consent based on sound understanding in order to allow an informed choice prior to any intervention and that their rights in decision-making and consent will be respected and upheld.

*continued overleaf . . .*

*continued . . .*

*By the first progression point:*

i.   Seeks consent prior to sharing confidential information outside of the professional care team, subject to agreed safeguarding and protection procedures.

*By the second progression point:*

iii.   Ensures that the meaning of consent to treatment and care is understood by the people or service users.

*By entry to the register:*

vii.   Demonstrates respect for the autonomy and rights of people to withhold consent in relation to treatment within legal frameworks and in relation to people's safety.

## Chapter aims

By the end of this chapter, you should be able to:

*   explain ethical sensitivity in nurses' decision-making;
*   identify and apply ethical principles to nursing practice;
*   relate the NMC Code to nurses' duties in decision-making;
*   discuss topical ethical issues and dilemmas in nursing;
*   appreciate that ethical values affect all nursing decisions.

# Introduction

This chapter discusses **ethical sensitivity in decision-making**. As nurses we are duty bound to abide by a professional and ethical code of conduct (NMC, 2008) at all times, so in effect each decision we make has to be ethically justifiable. Ethical sensitivity in decision-making involves applying moral values and ethical principles in caring for patients, their families, and the public.

For the purposes of this chapter the following understanding of the term is adopted:

> *Ethical sensitivity in decision-making is applying ethical principles (patients' freedom of choice, actions should benefit not harm them, and fairness to all) in respecting patients' dignity and confidentiality, enabling their informed consent, and resolving moral dilemmas in nursing care.*

In this chapter we explore the theory and practice of ethical sensitivity in decision-making by: discussing and applying relevant RCN principles of nursing practice; exploring the philosophical basis and influence on clinical decision-making of different ethical theories; and summarising ethical principles in healthcare and relating them to the Code (NMC, 2008). We also outline how moral and ethical considerations are incorporated in law. Case studies and learning activities highlighting ethical issues and dilemmas when caring for patients help to link theory and practice throughout the chapter. Finally, the strengths and weaknesses of ethical sensitivity in nurses' clinical decision-making are summarised.

# Ethical sensitivity in RCN principles of nursing practice

The RCN (2010) has listed eight principles of nursing practice on their website accompanied by six video clips giving evidence of how they have been applied in caring for real patients (see **www.rcn.org.uk/development/practice/principles/story_wall**). We will select and refer to the nursing practice principles that flag up ethical issues, for example, enabling a person to die peacefully and with dignity. This is especially challenging and heart-rending when the dying patient is a child, as illustrated by the following case study, which is a written version of one of the video clips. The dignity, bravery and maturity of the young child in the case study is remarkable, and you are asked to reflect on the ethical sensitivity shown in her care during the first five activities.

## Case study: 10 going on 80

*Habib, an interpreter, is reflecting upon his involvement in the care of Yasmin, a terminally ill ten-year-old girl whose family immigrated to the UK from Pakistan. Habib's main role is to enable communication between Yasmin, her family and the doctors and nurses. In this particular instance his role is to convey Yasmin's last wishes to her father. Habib explains that Yasmin has received medical treatment for most of her young life. She is very small for her age, almost blind, partially deaf, has poor control of her bowels, and her kidneys are failing. Habib describes Yasmin as '10 going on 80' as she seems to have such a wise head on such young shoulders in living her severely restricted life to the full, inspiring admiration and respect from everyone who knows her, and in facing up to the inevitability of her own premature death.*

*Yasmin is cared for in a hospital unit. One day she creates an opportunity to talk to Habib in private by asking her dad to fetch her some clothes, and while he's away she asks Habib to sit down as she needs to ask him something. Yasmin explains she knows she is going to die soon and when that happens she would like Habib to tell her dad she wants to be buried in Pakistan, next to her grandfather, with all her toys as she doesn't want anyone else to play with them. She says it is difficult for her to talk directly to her dad about this. About a week later Yasmin's health deteriorates and she whispers to Habib to remind him of her request. Sometime later Yasmin dies. Habib tells her dad what she has said. He replies, 'I was going to do that anyway, I loved her.'*

*(Adapted from RCN, 2010)*

Although Habib is not a nurse, his role as an interpreter gives him temporary membership of the healthcare team and also of Yasmin's extended family, both of which are concerned with caring for her. Habib responds to Yasmin's request in a way we as nurses might, and this is why the RCN suggest that the case study helps to illustrate the following principles of nursing practice:

*Principle A*
*Nurses and nursing staff treat everyone in their care with dignity and humanity – they understand their individual needs, show compassion and sensitivity, and provide care that respects all people equally.*

*Principle D*
*Nurses and nursing staff provide and promote care that puts people at the centre, involves patients, service users, their families and their carers in decisions and helps them make informed choices about their treatment and care.*
(RCN, 2010, p1)

Now you have read the case study and principles A and D, you are ready to tackle Activity 9.1.

---

### Activity 9.1            *Evidence-based practice and research*

In using video clips of practitioners' reflections on patient care, the RCN offers evidence to support its principles of nursing practice. This activity encourages you to look more closely at the evidence (case study information derived from the video clip) and decide whether it does or does not support the principles the RCN associates with it. See if you can identify examples where Habib appeared to apply principles A and D (or not). Do you agree or disagree with the RCN that Habib demonstrated effective application of the principles? Please explain the reasons for your judgement using examples from the case study.

*Some possible answers are included at the end of the chapter.*

---

In undertaking Activity 9.1, you make a start at probing and understanding how ethical considerations are part and parcel of everyday healthcare interventions. In RCN principles A and D, the references to dignity, humanity, compassion, sensitivity, respect, equality, patient-centred care, and informed choice reflect the application of moral values and ethical sensitivity in decision-making. This involves translating caring qualities associated with nurses into clinical decision-making and subsequent actions that are humane and professionally competent, that empower patients to be active participants, and that achieve the best possible care outcomes.

Maintaining confidentiality, dealing with patients' or relatives' complaints, and reporting nurses' concerns about standards of care also involve applying moral values and ethical sensitivity in decision-making. This point is supported by another of the RCN principles:

*Principle E*
*Nurses and nursing staff are at the heart of the communication process: they assess, record and report on treatment and care, handle information sensitively and confidentially, deal with complaints effectively, and are conscientious in reporting the things they are concerned about.*
(RCN, 2010, p1)

The RCN website does not link principle E with Habib's story, but Activity 9.2 asks you to do so.

---

**Activity 9.2**                                          *Decision-making*

Principle E is applicable to the case study since Habib was *at the heart of the communication process* regarding Yasmin's care, he appeared to *handle information sensitively* when Yasmin effectively told him her 'last will and testament', and he treated this information *confidentially* and only disclosed the details to Yasmin's dad after her death, as she had requested. In order to dig deeper at ethical issues regarding Habib's decision-making, please answer the following:

1. If you were in Habib's place, would you have acted in the same way or not? Please explain why you would or would not or suggest what else you might have done.
2. Do you think Habib was right to keep Yasmin's wishes confidential until after she died as she had requested? If so, why? If not, why not?
3. If someone argues that Habib's actions were wrong because they might encourage vulnerable young girls to share secrets with unrelated grown men, how would you respond to this?
4. Given that when Habib told Yasmin's dad how she wanted to be buried, he said he was going to do that anyway, did Habib actually achieve anything by telling him? If so, what?
5. Imagine Habib is on leave when Yasmin dies and her dad does not know what she said. Now suppose he buries her in the UK, not Pakistan, so he can visit her more often. What potential ethical issues arise from this situation, and how could they have been avoided?

*Some possible answers can be found at the end of the chapter.*

---

Activity 9.2 gives you a taste of how to question, defend or perhaps amend decision-making in relation to its possible ethical justification. In order to understand and explain ethical issues in more depth it is helpful to look at relevant philosophical perspectives.

# Philosophical basis of ethical sensitivity in decision-making

Philosophy is an advanced type of critical thinking seeking answers to questions about the meaning of human existence, nature of knowledge, moral values, political organisation and desirable behaviour. The study of ethics is a branch of philosophy, and different philosophers emphasise the importance of different priorities in ethical theory, as briefly outlined in Table 9.1.

## Virtues

Aristotle focused on the importance of people developing a virtuous character, which he thought led to personal wisdom, happiness and a strong community. He named it 'Nicomachean' ethics

| Ethical focus | Virtues | Rights and duties | Outcomes |
|---|---|---|---|
| Defining morality | Being a good person | Doing good things | Getting good results |
| Examples applying ethical priorities | Honesty, caring, fair-minded, brave | Get informed consent before treating patient | Healthcare problem is satisfactorily resolved |
| Questioning and evaluating conduct | Would a reasonable person act the same way in the situation? | Did the nurse act in accordance with NMC code of conduct? | Do benefits of care outweigh the costs to patient or to society? |
| Corresponding ethical theories | Nicomachean (how to develop a good character) | Deontology (theoretical principles of moral duties) | Consequentialism and utilitarianism (maximising benefits) |
| Philosopher linked to ethical theory | Aristotle (384–322 BC) | Immanuel Kant (1724–1804) | Jeremy Bentham (1748–1832) |

*Table 9.1: Virtues, rights and duties, and outcomes in ethical theories*

after his son Nicomachus, reinforcing the view that developing good character is a consequence of lifelong learning and practising the right habits with input from parents, teachers and scholars.

Despite being over 2,000 years old, Aristotle's focus on human virtues remains very influential; nursing students have to demonstrate that they are of 'good character'; for example, they must not have any criminal conviction – to protect the public from those deemed morally unfit to practice (NMC, 2009a). Similarly, if you look at the Essential Skills Clusters box at the start of the chapter you can see each one begins with *People can trust a newly registered graduate* . . .. Honesty and trustworthiness are human virtues like those Aristotle associated with ethical conduct. Evaluating appropriateness of behaviour according to whether a reasonable person would have acted similarly in same situation (Table 9.1) is still used as a guide to dispense legal and moral justice. In Activity 9.2, question 1 invited you to test this out by putting yourself in Habib's shoes and deciding whether or not you would have acted in the same way. Courage or bravery is another useful virtue for nurses to possess to cope with physical, emotional and mental demands that many people might find difficult or feel squeamish about. The case study also showed that we can often learn a lot from patients in this respect, given Yasmin's remarkable fortitude in suffering serious illness most of her short life, and facing her fears about dying with such dignity.

# Rights and duties

Good personal qualities or virtues such as caring are essential in nursing, but more concrete and specific guidance is needed in applying ethical principles to policies, procedures and decision-making. This is where Kant's deontological theory comes into play since we need to know what patients' rights are so we can make it our duty to respect those rights in our dealings with them. They are referred to in NMC *Standards for pre-registration nursing education* under 'professional values', for example, *empower [people to make] choices that promote self-care and safety* (first box, start of chapter). It is reinforced in the Essential Skills Clusters (second box, start of chapter), such as: *empowering people to make choices; gain their consent . . . prior to any intervention; seeks consent prior to sharing confidential information;* and *people's rights in decision-making and consent will be respected and upheld.* Professional and ethical principles in nursing (NMC, 2008) can also be used to both guide and evaluate nurses' conduct (Table 9.1). In investigating any complaints about registered nurses a panel appointed by the NMC will also refer to the Code in deciding whether it has been breached, and if the nurse remains fit to practise or not.

In the case study Yasmin appeared empowered, taking the initiative to ask Habib to convey her burial wishes to her dad after she died. It is unlikely Yasmin would have done this unless she trusted Habib, and he honoured that trust by telling her dad what she said. In Activity 9.2, questions 2 and 3 asked you to think about potential ethical implications of Habib keeping his agreement with Yasmin confidential until the time came to reveal what she said. It helps to show that ethical dilemmas can occur where seemingly opposing duties (empowering self-determination of patients while safeguarding vulnerable minors) need addressing. Resolving dilemmas is a judgement call, and it is advisable to involve other healthcare team members (not doing so leaves the practitioner vulnerable to accusations if something goes wrong). If a child is involved, we would normally include parents but in this case it was against Yasmin's wishes, as she did not feel the time was right for her dad to know what she was thinking about. In the RCN's video clip it does not say whether Habib discussed Yasmin's wishes with healthcare team before he told her dad or not. Activity 9.2 assumed the latter; Activity 9.3 assumes the former.

## Activity 9.3 — *Team working*

However good a rapport we have established with a patient, we are part of a team with whom responsibility for care is shared. Communicating significant developments to members of the team is therefore important in order for care to be well informed, responsive to changes, coordinated and consistent. This activity asks you to imagine that Habib wants to get Yasmin's consent for him to share her wishes with the team. Please answer the following questions.

1. What are the advantages of sharing the information with the healthcare team?
2. What anxieties might Yasmin have about agreeing to this?
3. If you were in Habib's place, what would you say to inform Yasmin's decision in consenting (or not consenting) to sharing with the team the information she had told you in confidence?
4. If Yasmin is in agreement, what duty of care would team members have in this respect?
5. If Yasmin does not consent to sharing information with the team, what would you do?

*Some possible answers can be found at the end of the chapter.*

# Outcomes

Being of good character, respecting patients' rights, and fulfilling our professional duties may contribute to good outcomes of care, but ultimately, the success of care is judged by whether the patient's health improves, deteriorates, or does not change. Working towards achieving good outcomes for patients is also referred to in the following RCN principle of nursing practice:

*Principle G*
*Nurses and nursing staff work closely with their own team and with other professionals, making sure patients' care is co-ordinated, is of a high standard and has the best possible outcome.*
(RCN, 2010, p1)

This is where ethical theories of consequentialism or utilitarianism are relevant since they focus on outcomes. NMC professional values (see the box at the start of the chapter) apply them to underline the importance of achieving outcomes that assure patients' safety while they *manage risk and promote health and well-being*. Hence, both consequentialism and utilitarianism emphasise that actions are morally good if the outcomes indicate that things have improved (Table 9.1).

Conversely, actions are morally suspect if things get worse (even if the correct procedures have been followed). This approach can be described as the 'ends justifying the means', which is in direct contrast to rights and duties, which focus more on following the correct procedures or the 'means justifying the ends'. The main difference between consequentialism and utilitarianism is that the latter asserts that outcomes that benefit the greatest number of people are better than those that benefit one or two people. Utilitarianism may therefore be used to link ethics with social theory, politics and economics (e.g. funding more cost-effective treatments so that more people can benefit, while rationing less cost-effective treatments). Activity 9.4 is intended to help you to clarify the differences between these two 'outcomes focused' ethical theories.

---

## Activity 9.4 — *Reflection*

Read the following moral assumptions regarding Yasmin's care and identify whether you think they are describing the application of consequentialism or utilitarianism, and explain why.

1. It is wrong in today's day and age, with all the medical and scientific knowledge at our disposal, that more was not done to prolong Yasmin's life (we are not told why a kidney transplant that might have enabled her to survive longer was not performed).

2. It is wrong in today's financial climate that so many resources were used to fight a losing battle in keeping Yasmin alive for so long when the money could have saved many more lives by tackling preventable causes of death, for example by increasing the uptake of immunisations against childhood diseases and supervising children at risk of non-accidental injuries.

3. It is right that the healthcare team helped Yasmin to gain a few more years of life (which she truly appreciated and made the most of) than she would have had without their help.

*continued opposite . . .*

---

*continued . . .*

4. It is right that the healthcare team helped Yasmin to gain a few more years of life because in doing so they learnt more about her disease and how to treat it, so the knowledge and expertise will be invaluable in contributing to more effective care of other similar children.

*Some possible answers can be found at the end of the chapter.*

Activity 9.4 looked at alternative perspectives of whether outcomes of Yasmin's medical care were successful or unsuccessful. Earlier, in Activity 9.2, questions 4 and 5, you explored the outcomes of Habib conveying or not conveying Yasmin's wishes to her dad as promised. In Activity 9.5 you are asked to apply consequentialism and utilitarianism to Habib's actions.

## Activity 9.5          *Reflection*

Read the following moral assumptions regarding Habib's actions and identify if you think they are describing the application of consequentialism or utilitarianism. Explain why.

1. Habib was wrong not to tell the healthcare team about Yasmin's request because if anything had happened to him no one else could have told her dad what she said.
2. Habib was wrong not to tell the healthcare team about Yasmin's request because they needed to know what was worrying her to be sensitive to her needs in the last weeks of her life, and also to inform their understanding and care of other children in the future.
3. Habib was right to agree to Yasmin's request because it helped ease her fears about dying to think she would have all her toys with her and be buried next to her grandfather, and it saved her from talking about it with her dad, which she did not feel able to do.
4. Habib was right to agree to Yasmin's request because it not only benefited her, it also comforted her dad and family to know they were doing what she wanted, and, in telling Yasmin's story, Habib helped many nurses value ethical sensitivity in decision-making.

*Some possible answers can be found at the end of the chapter.*

Both Activity 9.4 and 9.5 highlight the debatable nature of the rights and wrongs of actions and their consequences. In other words, ethical decisions are never 'cut and dried'; there is always an element of uncertainty in wondering if the right decision has been made, and this makes them the most challenging decisions healthcare professionals have to deal with. We have seen that outcomes of healthcare can be interpreted differently as right or wrong, according to the moral assumptions or ethical perspective that is applied. As a general rule of thumb, when we are focusing on getting the best outcomes for a particular patient we are applying consequentialism, and when we are focusing on the bigger picture in getting the best outcomes for all potential patients and the public at large we are applying utilitarianism.

In this section we have used relevant moral philosophy to describe personal qualities (virtues), theoretical principles (rights and duties), and practical benefits (outcomes) associated with ethical sensitivity in clinical decision-making. As nurses we have to combine and apply all of these different strands to be the best person that we can be, provide the best care possible, and achieve the best results for patients. In the next section we explore some of the challenges in applying ethical principles and the NMC Code in delivering high standards of care to patients.

# Applying ethical principles and the NMC Code in decision-making

| Ethical principles | Relevant extracts: the Code (NMC, 2008) |
|---|---|
| AUTONOMY<br>Respect service users' right of self-determination and freedom of choice | *You must respect people's right to confidentiality* (p2); *You must listen to the people in your care and respond to their concerns and preferences* (p3); *You must share with people, in a way they can understand, the information they want or need to know about their health* (p3); *You must ensure you gain consent before you begin any treatment or care* (p4); *You must respect and support people's rights to accept or decline treatment and care* (p4); *You must uphold people's rights to be fully involved in decisions about their care* (p4). |
| NON-MALEFICENCE<br>Do not cause service users any harm (first principle of First-Aid) | *You must disclose information if you believe someone may be at risk of harm* (p2); *You must act without delay if you believe that you, a colleague or anyone else may be putting someone at risk* (p6); *You must report your concerns in writing if problems in the environment of care are putting people at risk* (p6); *You must act immediately to put matters right if someone in your care has suffered harm for any reason* (p9). |
| BENEFICENCE<br>Enable service users to achieve best possible state of health and sense of wellbeing | *You must be able to demonstrate that you have acted in someone's best interest if you have provided care in an emergency* (p4); *You must work with colleagues to monitor the quality of your work and maintain the safety of those in your care* (p5); *You must make a referral to another practitioner when it is in the best interests of someone in your care* (p5); *You must deliver care based on the available evidence or best practice* (p7). |
| JUSTICE<br>Be fair-minded, treat service users equally in matching care delivery to their respective needs | *You must not discriminate in any way against those in your care* (p2); *You must make arrangements to meet people's language and communication needs* (p3); *You must treat your colleagues fairly and without discrimination* (p5); *You must demonstrate a personal and professional commitment to equality and diversity* (p9); *You must not allow someone's complaint to prejudice the care you provide for them* (p9); *You must not abuse your privileged position for your own ends* (p10). |

*Table 9.2: Autonomy, non-maleficence, beneficence, justice and the NMC Code*

The Code (NMC, 2008) specifies the professional and ethical requirements to practice as a registered nurse. Many of these reflect aspects of moral philosophy and associated ethical principles discussed earlier. If you find the theory a bit difficult to grasp, you do not have to worry too much because as long as you abide by the Code you will be applying ethical principles to practice. Four key ethical principles have been derived from moral philosophy and these are thought to capture the essential virtues, rights and duties, and outcomes that, as nurses, we should always strive to achieve in caring for patients. The four ethical principles are *autonomy, non-maleficence, beneficence* and *justice* (Beauchamp and Childress, 1989). Table 9.2 cross-references them with relevant extracts of the Code to help link ethical theory to practice.

# Autonomy and beneficence

The principle of autonomy or self-determination underpins Orem's self-care model (Chapter 1) where nurses continually assess what patients can or cannot do for themselves and help them with the latter (beneficence). It is also intrinsic to collaborative clinical decision-making (Chapter 2) where patients actively participate in and influence the nursing decisions that affect them. In the following case study a well-informed, articulate patient is unable to persuade a nurse of the seriousness of her symptoms, and this contributes to the ensuing fatal consequences.

## Case study: Fobbed off

*One weekend Miranda, aged 26, woke up with swelling and pain in her calf. She waited until Thursday to see if it would go away. When it did not she looked at a symptom checker for leg pain on the NHS Direct website and answered a series of questions. It indicated she might have a blood clot – deep vein thrombosis (DVT) in her calf and advised Miranda to see her GP and to take painkillers as needed. The earliest appointment offered was the next Monday (four days' time). Miranda was concerned about the delay in seeing the GP. She was anxious because she remembered her mum had had a DVT at the age of 21 and she thought this might increase her risk of having one. She also took contraceptive pills that increased her risk of blood clots. Miranda took aspirin both for the pain and because she knew it was supposed to help thin the blood.*

*On Friday, Miranda was so worried about her leg that she attended an NHS walk-in centre where she explained her concerns to Judy, an experienced nurse. Judy did not agree with Miranda's view and advised her to go home and rest as it was probably a muscle strain. Afterwards, she cried as she spoke to her husband on the phone, telling him she'd been 'fobbed off'. Miranda did not see her GP on the Monday because on the Sunday she collapsed and died from a pulmonary embolism (blood clot in the lung), a known fatal complication associated with having an underlying DVT.*

*(Adapted from 'Woman dies after being "fobbed off"' by Chris Brooke,* Daily Mail, *20 October 2010)*

The case study is a disturbing account of what can happen when a service user's autonomy is disregarded. Through her resourcefulness and intelligence Miranda managed to piece things together and come up with the correct provisional diagnosis. All she needed was a healthcare professional to emulate what she had done (or refer her to someone who could) so that she could receive the right investigations and treatment. Tragically, this was not to be. There are many aspects of the case study that go beyond the scope of this chapter: Was the NHS Direct advice appropriate? Why couldn't the GP see her sooner? How far away was the main Accident and Emergency centre? We will focus here on Miranda's contact with Judy, the nurse at the NHS walk-in centre. Activity 9.6 asks you some questions regarding this.

---

## Activity 9.6                                  *Leadership and management*

Imagine that you are a lay member on a clinical governance committee at the NHS Trust where Miranda died. Your job is to represent the interests of service users. You are concerned about Judy's inability to do an accurate risk assessment. This has implications for better supervision and continuing professional development of all nurses. You decide to read the Code (NMC, 2008) to see what registered nurses are supposed to do. You identify requirements that, had they been complied with, Judy might have acted differently, with a better outcome for Miranda.

Please read through the case study and the NMC extracts associated with autonomy and beneficence in Table 9.2 once again, before answering the following questions.

1.  Which NMC requirements of registered nurses to respect or empower patient autonomy appeared to be lacking or needed improving in the case study and why?
2.  Which NMC requirements of registered nurses to apply beneficence within high quality patient care appeared to be lacking or needed improving in the case study and why?
3.  What recommendations would you make to improve the NHS Trust's walk-in service?

*Some possible answers can be found at the end of the chapter.*

---

Activity 9.6 highlights the importance of registered nurses reading and practising the Code in order to effectively apply the ethical principles of autonomy and beneficence. In the next case study a district nurse offers an elderly lady a higher level of care than she actually wants.

---

### Case study: Choosing to live alone

*Margaret, aged 81, is a widow who lives alone in a council flat where she has lived for 35 years. Ten years ago she had a stroke, leaving her with muscle weakness and blind in one eye. She also has arthritis, late onset diabetes and difficulty controlling her bladder. Margaret takes tablets for arthritis, blood pressure and diabetes, and wears a pad in case of 'accidents'. She is visited regularly by three daughters who cook for her and ensure she has the right diet. Margaret lives on the fourth floor and there is no lift. She has not been out of her flat for six years when her son-in-law, who used to help carry her up and down the stairs, had to stop after having a heart attack.*

*continued opposite . . .*

*continued . . .* •••••••••••••••••••••••••••••••••••••••••••••••••••••••••••••••••••••••••••••••

> *Elizabeth, a district nurse, has known Margaret since she had the stroke and over the years has coordinated the supply of a walking frame and adaptations in the flat to help her get around, including a sit-in bath, a raised toilet seat, hand rails in the corridor, a Stena chair lift in the short stairway from the living area to bedrooms, and an emergency buzzer system she can call for help with. Her family also bought a special armchair, which electronically helps her to sit, elevate feet and stand up. Margaret's mobility has deteriorated recently and she has had a number of falls. Her daughters ask Elizabeth to assess Margaret's safety as they believe she now needs constant care and supervision. When Elizabeth sees Margaret she explains that it is possible for her to move to a residential home nearby where she will be looked after on the ground floor so she can get out in the garden (she loves flowers and has lots of pots on her balcony) and the girls can visit as they do now. She tells Margaret that the GP has said he would be happy to support such a referral, and it seems that her daughters believe this is the safest and best thing for her also. Margaret tells Elizabeth she does not want to move, that she loves her flat, and that when the time comes she wants 'to die in my own home'. Elizabeth accepts Margaret's decision and increases her visits to monitor her health and help Margaret exercise and strengthen her legs.*

In this case study, Elizabeth appears to be well aware of the health risks and how these can be controlled, while also respecting Margaret's preferences. In Activity 9.7 you are asked to consider how she was able to achieve this.

## Activity 9.7 — *Decision-making*

With reference to the case study and relevant NMC extracts (in Table 9.2), describe how Elizabeth balanced and applied the ethical principles of autonomy and beneficence in Margaret's care.

1. Following Margaret's stroke.
2. In responding to her daughters' request for an urgent assessment.
3. When Margaret declined the residential care option.

*Some possible answers can be found at the end of the chapter.*

Activity 9.7 highlights a constant tension between respecting someone's freedom of choice and providing the best possible care. Ethical sensitivity in decision-making is therefore challenging, and requires the integration and application of a range of relevant knowledge skills and attitudes. Table 9.3 illustrates this regarding the care Elizabeth provided for Margaret.

Table 9.3 also shows how the conceptions of nursing complement application of ethical principles (autonomy and beneficence) in decision-making. Beneficence and non-maleficence are 'opposite sides of the same coin', the former maximising helpful, the latter minimising harmful outcomes of nursing care. In practice many healthcare interventions, while being helpful, can also have less helpful or sometimes harmful outcomes; for example, antibiotics save lives most of the time but if someone is allergic to them they can be life-threatening. It is vital to make sure that benefits of care outweigh costs to each patient's health and well-being. Applying non-maleficence requires

| Conceptions of nursing | Ethical sensitivity in decision-making |
|---|---|
| Caring | Committing to maximising Margaret's health and well-being |
| Listening and being there | Responding to daughters' worries and Margaret's wishes |
| Practical procedures | Providing exercises to increase strength/flexibility of Margaret's legs |
| Knowledge and understanding | Understanding risks posed by medical problems and Margaret's frailty |
| Communicating | Explaining to Margaret possible benefits of residential care |
| Patience | Allowing Margaret time to decide what she wants to do |
| Teamwork | Liaising with GP/council/social services to get flat adapted |
| Paperwork and electronic record | Writing up risk assessment, recommendations and action |
| Empathising and non-judgemental | Understanding Margaret's reluctance to move out of her flat |
| Professional | Applying NMC Code to treat Margaret with dignity and respect |

*Table 9.3: Integrating ethical sensitivity in decision-making and conceptions of nursing*

vigilance in order to avoid making costly mistakes through carelessness or ignorance. This is why in first-aid training you are first taught not to harm the victim. This may seem obvious, but if you do not know what you are doing, it can often do more harm than good.

# Non-maleficence and justice

Ethical principles of non-maleficence and justice often to go together in healthcare because it is unfair for service users to be harmed rather than helped by those they trust to take care of them. One of the areas nurses have to be particularly careful about is the administration of medicines, including checking if it is the right drug, right dose, right route, right person, every time. This is especially important in caring for young children, who need much smaller doses than adults. In the next case study the nurses do not follow procedure properly, with fatal consequences.

## Case study: Tragic outcome of misreading prescription

*Max was born prematurely, weighing less than two pounds. He needed intensive treatment in a high dependency neonatal unit to enable him to survive. After three months he weighed over six pounds and was thought strong enough to undergo necessary abdominal surgery. Some time after the operation Max was prescribed an intravenous solution of 5ml of sodium chloride in 1 litre of fluid to ensure he was adequately hydrated and to maintain the correct sodium level. Instead of 5ml the ward manager and the staff nurse checking and administering the solution put 50ml (ten times the prescribed dose) of sodium chloride by mistake. The overdose led to Max being severely dehydrated. He lost weight, suffered brain damage, and died when he was only four months old.*

*(Adapted from 'First picture of baby who died after suspected salt overdose from hospital drip' by Caroline Grant,* Daily Mail, *24 July 2009)*

The case study graphically demonstrates the importance of vigilance in giving medicines and the danger of complacency in not carefully reading and checking prescriptions. The 'failsafe' system failed. The nurse whose role it was to check what the other was doing should have spotted the discrepancy between what was prescribed and what was being administered and acted promptly to stop her colleague (see 'Non-maleficence' NMC extracts in Table 9.2). All the good work the neonatal unit had done was undone by two nurses' lack of vigilance, with tragic results. It underlines the earlier point that a nurse's first duty is not to harm patients. In Activity 9.8 you are asked to reflect on the implications of the case study in your own area of practice.

### Activity 9.8 — *Reflection*

As a nursing student you will be asked to help administer medication, including checking if it is the right drug/dose/route for the right patient. You cannot do this safely and effectively unless you understand what the drugs are for, their optimal therapeutic dose, side effects and possible contraindications (people who should avoid them). Think about the medicines patients receive in your current or previous practice placement and look up the ones you are unsure of (use the current version of the *British National Formulary*). Try to make connections between each patient's health problems and their prescribed medicine so that you know why the patient needs it, how it works, and what to watch out for. Do not forget to consider each patient's body weight and how that might affect the prescribed dosage, especially in relation to children. This can help to make what might otherwise seem a routine task more meaningful, and by prompting you to question what you are doing it also helps to reduce errors.

*As this is for your own reflection, there is no outline answer provided.*

Activity 9.8 and the previous case study suggest that although nurses' first instinct may be to do things to help people (beneficence), they need to counter-balance this by continually assessing health risks they may pose to patients themselves and reducing these (non-maleficence). Sometimes harm suffered by patients is more psychological than physical, resulting from stereotyping, prejudice or a lack of understanding, as the next case study illustrates.

## Case study: A patient wants to smoke

*Joanne, a third-year nursing student, was reflecting on an incident that occurred during her last practice placement in an acute medical ward. Katia, aged 25, an Estonian tourist visiting London, had collapsed and been admitted to Joanne's ward for observation and investigation. Katia had regained consciousness, but she spoke very little English and communication was difficult. She had an intravenous infusion in her arm to aid hydration. No one knew exactly what was wrong with her because the results of blood tests and other investigations were not yet known. Some HCAs said she was a 'manipulative patient' because she talked 'in her own language', kept wanting to go out of the ward for a cigarette, and pulled her intravenous infusion out when no one helped her carry it outside so that she could have a smoke. When the staff nurse saw what Katia had done she shouted at her and then Katia threw a jug of water at the staff nurse. Joanne thought that Katia was confused, frightened and frustrated that she had no one she could talk to. By the end of the day Katia was transferred to the mental health unit where it was felt they would be better able to manage her 'violent behaviour'.*

The case study suggests that nurses and HCAs may not always be as caring, non-judgemental and empathising as the conceptions of nursing (in Table 9.3) advocate. Activity 9.9 asks you to apply the ethical principle of justice in reviewing what happened in the case study.

### Activity 9.9 *Communication*

Many of the difficulties described in the case study arose from a lack of communication between Katia and the ward staff. Refer to the relevant NMC extracts associated with the ethical principle of justice in Table 9.2 when answering the following questions.

1. Which of the NMC requirements were not addressed in the treatment of Katia?
2. Was it fair or unfair for the HCAs to refer to Katia as a 'manipulative patient'?
3. What could the staff have done to facilitate better communication with Katia?
4. Was it fair or unfair to call Katia 'violent' and move her to a mental health unit?
5. In what way did Joanne differ from her colleagues in her assessment of Katia?

*Some possible answers can be found at the end of the chapter.*

Activity 9.9 and the previous case study focus on the ethical principle of justice or fairness. Just as we are duty bound to avoid harming patients (non-maleficence), we are also obligated to address biases, stereotypes and prejudices that can lead us to treat others unfairly. Until we can achieve this we will never be able to treat all people fairly or as equals. This is not easy to achieve if nurses are stressed, and the extra demands required by some patients exposes them as feeling 'burnt out' and unable to cope. An increase in violence against nurses and other healthcare staff in Accident and Emergency centres can compound perceived stress and highlight that nurses also need to be protected. Ultimately, justice is dispensed through legislation, and in the final section we look briefly at how respecting and addressing moral and ethical principles is, in fact, a legal obligation.

# How moral and ethical considerations are incorporated in law

The virtues, rights and duties, and outcomes we discussed earlier are not confined to texts on moral philosophy. Similarly, ethical principles of autonomy, non-maleficence, beneficence and justice are not confined to university lecture theatres. Throughout the chapter, with reference to topical case studies, we have shown how these ideas can help to distinguish between good and poor nursing practice to maximise the former and minimise the latter. These principles are not confined to nursing, as they are incorporated within British and European law as basic human rights and duties that everyone is both entitled to and bound to abide by. The impetus for this came in the wake of revelations about atrocities in the Second World War. In the UK we are protected by the Human Rights Act 1998, which reflects each of the ethical principles (shown in brackets) that we discussed earlier, as follows.

- *The right to life* (beneficence).
- *Freedom from torture and degrading treatment* (non-maleficence).
- *The right to liberty* (autonomy).
- *The right to respect for private and family life* (autonomy).
- *Freedom of thought, conscience and religion, and freedom to express your beliefs* (autonomy).
- *The right not to be discriminated against in respect of these rights and freedoms* (justice).

If we feel our rights are infringed, we can seek justice under the terms of the Human Rights Act. For example, in September 2010 a 16-stone woman argued that an NHS Trust denied her human rights by refusing to do a gastric bypass operation to help her to lose weight. The court agreed with her. Furthermore, if any party is unhappy with the court's judgement, they are entitled to appeal to the European Court of Human Rights. Hence the ethical theories that we have discussed are endorsed by philosophers, the RCN, the NMC, and UK and European legal systems.

### Chapter summary

In this chapter we defined ethical sensitivity in decision-making and explored its origins and applications. We identified ethical values in the RCN's principles of nursing practice and explored their philosophical basis in terms of being good, doing good and good outcomes. Four key ethical principles were identified – autonomy, non-maleficence, beneficence and justice – and they were cross-referenced to relevant extracts of the NMC code of conduct. It was noted that these ethical principles are also applied within the Human Rights Act 1988. Autonomy and beneficence were related to the conceptions of nursing identified in

*continued overleaf . . .*

*continued . . .*

previous chapters showing how they complement one another. The strengths of this approach are in translating nurses' caring qualities into ethical sensitivity within decision-making that is humane, professionally competent, empowers patients to be active participants, and achieves the best possible care outcomes. The weaknesses of this approach are that it is complex, protracted and contentious, rarely reaching a definitive decision. Topical, often poignant case studies were integrated within the chapter to link theory and practice, and activities invited you to grapple with key issues.

## Activities: brief outline answers

### Activity 9.1 Evidence-based practice and research (page 140)

You may have included the following points.

*Applying Principle A (dignity, humanity, compassion)* Habib respected Yasmin's courage and wisdom for one so young (10 going on 80) and was sensitive regarding her wishes. His interpreter role helped the family communicate with staff.

*Applying Principle D (involve service users, families in decisions)* Habib followed Yasmin's lead in discussing her preferred burial arrangements and when to tell her dad about her decision, so in effect, he allowed the service user to make use of him.

*Was Habib successful in applying Principle A and D?* Yes, because Yasmin appeared to trust him and he honoured that trust as outlined above.

### Activity 9.2 Decision-making (page 141)

You may have included the following points.

1.  Say yes if you would do same as Habib in order to ease Yasmin's fear about dying.
2.  Say yes if Habib was right to keep it confidential until the time came, as that was Yasmin's wish.
3.  Ordinarily it is unwise to encourage such secrets, but the circumstances were not ordinary. Yasmin initiated it, not Habib, and the reasons for not telling dad yet were understandable.
4.  Habib fulfilled his duty to Yasmin by telling her dad, and he learned her wishes would be met.
5.  The potential ethical consequences would be Habib not honouring his promise to Yasmin. It could have been avoided if he asked to be contacted or if he asked someone else to tell dad.

### Activity 9.3 Team working (page 143)

You may have included the following points.

1.  Improved communication, shared responsibility, back-up system if Habib not available.
2.  Yasmin may not know them so well, and might be worried they might tell her dad before the agreed time.
3.  Sharing information lessens risk of Yasmin's dad not knowing her wishes if Habib is away.
4.  Team members' duty of care to respect Yasmin's wishes about when to talk to her dad.
5.  If Yasmin does not consent, respect her wishes but make note in reflective journal or diary.

## Activity 9.4 Reflection (pages 144–5)

You may have included the following points.

1. Consequentialism – unable to save Yasmin's life.
2. Utilitarianism – unable to use money to save many other children's lives.
3. Consequentialism – managed to help Yasmin gain a few more years of life.
4. Utilitarianism – healthcare team gained knowledge they can use to treat other children.

## Activity 9.5 Reflection (page 145)

You may have included the following points.

1. Consequentialism – by not telling team they could not fulfil Yasmin's wish if Habib was away.
2. Utilitarianism – not telling team limits understanding so less well informed in caring for others.
3. Consequentialism – eased Yasmin's fears, saving her from talking to dad about her death.
4. Utilitarianism – Yasmin's story can help nurses apply ethical sensitivity with other patients.

## Activity 9.6 Leadership and management (page 148)

You may have included the following points:

1. 'Listen to the people in your care and respond to their concerns and preferences' and 'uphold people's rights to be fully involved in decisions about their care' (autonomy) need improving.
2. Application of all four NMC extracts re beneficence in Table 9.2 needs to be improved.
3. *Recommendations* Ensure nurses working in all emergency settings have the knowledge and skills to carry out accurate risk assessments; review management and supervision of walk-in centre personnel; ensure nurses are familiar with NMC Code and how to apply it within the specific clinical contexts in which they are practising; when patient refers to NHS Direct website symptom checker, use computer to check through questions and advice with them.

## Activity 9.7 Decision-making (page 149)

You may have included the following points.

1. Arranged for walking aid and adaptations to flat to help Margaret adjust to reduced vision and mobility, gave advice on medication and diet re diabetes, helped her to keep her home.
2. Undertook risk assessment regarding Margaret's frequent falls and deteriorating health and identified supervised residential care option and presented it to Margaret for her to decide.
3. Accepted Margaret's decision to decline residential care and increased home visits to give additional support and help her exercise and strengthen her legs.

## Activity 9.9 Communication (page 152)

You may have included the following points.

1. NMC justice requirements not met: *must not discriminate in any way against those in your care, must make arrangements to meet people's language and communication needs, must demonstrate a personal and professional commitment to equality and diversity.*
2. Unfair for HCAs to call Katia a 'manipulative patient' since they could not understand a word she spoke and could not, therefore, make that judgement unless it was based on prejudice.
3. Enable better communication by contacting interpreter, look up English–Estonian dictionary on the internet, give non-verbal gestures of support (smile), and avoid shouting at her.
4. Unfair for Katia to be labelled as 'violent' and moved to a mental health unit since the team have not managed to communicate with her to make an assessment of her mental health. It was wrong for her to throw the jug but she had just been shouted at in an unfriendly way. It is possible she might feel more

relaxed in the mental health unit where designated smoking areas are permitted for clients to use. Further medical treatment will depend on test results.

5. Joanne appeared to differ from the others because she put herself in Katia's place and tried to see things from her point of view as someone who is confused, frightened and frustrated.

## Further reading

**Griffith, R and Tengnah, C** (2010) *Law and Professional Issues in Nursing*, 2nd edition. Exeter: Learning Matters.

Helpful guide linking ethical principles with law and applying them to nursing practice.

**Fry, S and Johnstone, MJ** (2008) *Ethics in Nursing Practice: A guide to ethical decision-making*, 3rd edition. London: Blackwell Publishing.

First published by the International Council of Nurses, this book provides useful case studies on ethical decision-making.

## Useful websites

**www.rcn.org.uk/development/practice/principles**

Here you can find all eight RCN principles of nursing practice described and if you click link to 'story wall', you will find useful video clips.

**www.nursingtimes.net/nursing-practice**

Very informative website packed with wide ranging topical, ethical issues challenging nurses.

# Chapter 10
# Accountability for nursing decisions

*continued overleaf . . .*

*continued . . .*

> *By entry to the register:*
> ii.   Takes decisions and is able to answer for these decisions when required.
>
> 20.  People can trust the newly registered graduate nurse to select and manage medical devices safely.

## Chapter aims

By the end of this chapter, you should be able to:

- explain what accountability for nursing decisions means;
- identify different parties to whom nurses are accountable;
- understand ways in which accountability is applied in practice;
- discuss protective, deterrent, regulatory and educative functions;
- appreciate why nurses are accountable for all decisions, actions or omissions.

# Introduction

This chapter explores accountability for nursing decisions. We are held to account for what we do as nurses, at all times, and this is referred to in the Nurses and Midwives' Code of Conduct:

> *As a professional, you are personally accountable for actions and omissions in your practice and must always be able to justify your decisions.*
> (NMC, 2008, p1)

In the case study below a ward manager challenges a student nurse about his behaviour.

## Case study: Whistling in the treatment room

*Reggie is a first-year student on an adult nursing programme. While on placement in a medical ward he is shown how to dispose of used needles and syringes properly. Reggie has a habit of whistling tunes quite loudly when he is not working directly with the patients on the ward. One day, after giving an injection to a patient, under the supervision of his mentor, he is directed to dispose of the used needle and syringe in the treatment room. True to form, he starts whistling a tune rather loudly while alone in the treatment room. The ward manager can hear him while she is talking to a relative at the other end of the ward. She excuses herself for a moment to ask a staff nurse to go and tell Reggie to stop whistling.*

The case study shows how everything we do as nurses is open to scrutiny or criticism by others and may incur sanctions if our behaviour is deemed to be inappropriate. Activity 10.1 asks you to think about the case study a bit more as a way of beginning to explore nurses' accountability.

**Activity 10.1**                                    *Leadership and management*

In this activity you are asked to explore how nurses *must be able to justify decisions* (NMC, 2008) and reflect on what Reggie and the ward manager did by answering the following questions.

1.  Do you think Reggie was justified in whistling? If so, why?
2.  Do you think the ward manager was justified in stopping him from whistling? If so, why?

*Some possible answers can be found at the end of the chapter.*

Activity 10.1 illustrates a key feature of accountability: the need to justify decisions and actions we take as nurses (even seemingly innocuous activities such as whistling in the treatment room) because everything we do impacts upon patient care and the reputation of the profession. This chapter explores what accountability for nursing decisions means, who we are accountable to, how we are held to account, and why being accountable is so important in decision-making. In doing so we will understand how nurses' accountability fits into the bigger picture of NHS accountability, how it is applied in each of the decision-making styles discussed in previous chapters, the NMC's role regarding professional accountability, and how conceptions of nursing can be integrated and applied alongside accountability for nurses' clinical decision-making.

# What is accountability?

Accountability for nursing decisions requires us, at all times, to be able to give an account of what we are doing (or have done) to those to whom we are accountable. It involves describing or explaining decisions and resulting actions, justifying why they are or were necessary, and logically defending our decision-making processes and their outcomes when challenged to do so.

Accountability is a 'close cousin' of responsibility, with the latter associated with our particular roles as nurses and the various clinical activities we are expected to undertake. Nurses have always had many responsibilities in caring for patients, but it is only relatively recently that our professional autonomy has developed to a point where we are fully accountable for what we do. It requires a higher standard of education, which is why nursing is evolving into a graduate entry profession. Accountability is also linked to the development of evidence-based nursing practice because our decision-making and actions are more likely to be safe, effective and justifiable where they are supported by relevant research findings and principles of good practice. In the previous case study, the ward manager decided that Reggie's whistling was not justifiable. In the following case study a newly qualified nurse explains her understanding of accountability.

## Case study: Being responsible for nursing decisions

*Susan is in her first job as a staff nurse at a general hospital. In reflecting on the difference between being a student or a registered nurse she reveals her understanding of accountability.*

*'I've had to learn to think on my feet and make decisions on the spot. I need to be responsible and accountable for why I made those decisions. If someone asks why you are doing a certain procedure – like fitting anti-embolism stockings for a patient on bed rest to prevent the increased risk of deep vein thrombosis and pulmonary embolism – you need to be able to explain it is evidence-based and it works. You cannot just say, "because I'm the staff nurse!"'*

The case study illustrates how accountability means knowing how what you propose to do is of benefit to patients, and being able to explain it to them so that they understand and consent to it. In Activity 10.2 you are asked to think about your own examples in this respect.

## Activity 10.2                                           *Communication*

Think about your current or recent practice placements, and select three different examples of how you contributed to the care of patients. Did you do so because a colleague asked for help? Were you instructed to? Or did a patient ask you to help them? Describe what you did for the patient in each example. Then imagine that your link lecturer from the university asks you to explain the following.

- What were you doing for these patients?
- Were your actions of benefit to the patients and why?
- What evidence is there to support the effectiveness of your actions in caring for the patients?

Write down your responses to each of these questions. Discuss scenarios, questions and responses with a colleague, and take turns to question and explain to each other the rationale for decision-making and related nursing actions. It will give you practice in explaining your actions to others, which is at the heart of accountability for nursing decisions.

*As this is for your own reflection, there is no outline answer included for this activity.*

Activity 10.2 helps clarify what accountability for nursing decisions means using questions we need to ask ourselves (and be able to answer) when caring for patients. Of course, nurses do not care for patients in isolation from other healthcare professionals, most of whom are also employed by the NHS. The NHS is accountable for the organisation, management and delivery of a high standard of healthcare throughout the country, and our professional accountability as nurses therefore complements the goals of the NHS. Following an NHS review led by Lord Darzi (DH, 2008), principles and values were spelled out in an NHS Constitution for which all personnel (doctors, nurses, allied health professions, support services, managers) are accountable in applying. The constitution also identifies the responsibilities of service users in positively contributing to their own care. Table 10.1 summarises key principles and values of the new NHS Constitution.

| NHS principles | NHS values |
|---|---|
| 1. The NHS provides a comprehensive service available to all.<br>2. Access to NHS services is based on clinical need not an individual's ability to pay.<br>3. The NHS aspires to highest standards of excellence and professionalism.<br>4. NHS services must reflect the needs and preferences of patients, their families and their carers.<br>5. The NHS works across organisational boundaries and in partnerships with other organisations in the interest of patients, local communities and the wider population.<br>6. The NHS is committed to providing best value for taxpayers' money and the most effective, fair and sustainable use of finite resources<br>7. The NHS is accountable to the public, communities and patients that it serves | • *Everyone counts* (healthcare for all, no one is left out, and all have part to play in promoting and achieving personal and community health).<br>• *Compassion* (comfort and relieve suffering through being caring, kind and attentive).<br>• *Respect and dignity* (value each person as individual with own priorities, abilities, needs).<br>• *Working together for patients* (put needs of patients and communities first and overcome any restrictions of organisational boundaries).<br>• *Improving lives* (strive to improve health and well-being and people's experiences of NHS).<br>• *Commitment to quality of care* (earn trust by high standards of care – welcome feedback to learn from mistakes and build on successes). |

*Table 10.1: The NHS Constitution*

Source: Adapted from: Department of Health *The NHS Constitution* (for England) (DH, 2009)

The values identified in Table 10.1 complement those of nurses and other health professionals, and it is good to see that these are used to inform the principles of organising health services. The creation of the NHS Constitution was influenced by some well-publicised appalling instances of poor healthcare associated with poor management. This included being unresponsive to local needs while pursuing National Health targets, inadequate leadership regarding infection control, and lack of suitably qualified staff, facilities and equipment to cope with high clinical demands. Nurses and other health professionals are always personally accountable for the quality of care that they give, but if they are understaffed, under-resourced, poorly supervised and overworked, it is more difficult to maintain high standards. Recognising that patient needs and professional values should have more influence in structuring and managing services is vital in making NHS services more accountable to the needs of local communities. As nurses, we are accountable for upholding both our professional standards and principles and values of the NHS Constitution.

# Who are we accountable to?

First and foremost we are accountable to the patients, clients or service users to whom we owe a duty of care. We are accountable to the wider public, who indirectly pay for what we do via tax and national insurance. We are accountable to employers (e.g. the NHS), who enable our contact with patients by assigning us duties in employment contracts and job descriptions. Nurses are professionally accountable to the NMC to *provide a high standard of practice and care at all times* (NMC, 2008, p1). Like other citizens, we are accountable to society in abiding by civil law (e.g. Human Rights Act 1998: see Chapter 9) and criminal law (e.g. Theft Act 1968). Nursing students are also accountable to universities for their academic progress, and to clinical mentors or assessors who act as 'gatekeepers' to the profession in judging their professional suitability. Having clarified what accountability is and who we are accountable to we can define it thus:

> *Accountability in decision-making is being answerable to patients, public, employers, NMC and the law for the consequences of actions, and having to explain, justify and defend our decisions.*

# How do we demonstrate accountability?

In this section we will explore how we demonstrate accountability for nursing decisions through observation of our practice, record keeping, and all types and instances of our decision-making.

## Accountability and observation of our practice

Just as we use observation skills in assessing those in our care, we ourselves are continually observed by service users and members of the healthcare team. When we are attentive and responsive to patients' needs and preferences, we are demonstrating our accountability to them and they are more likely to feel well cared for and to evaluate the experience positively. If a patient is unhappy about the way we are caring for them, they are at liberty to make a complaint. We are then obliged to listen, apologise for any upset caused, and take action to remedy concerns. Sometimes healthcare colleagues act as advocates on behalf of patients (like the ward manager in the earlier case study) if they judge a team member's behaviour needs adjusting in patients' best interests. It is not always possible to have a team around you to observe, support and supervise what you are doing, for example, if you are nursing in community settings. Such nurses therefore need to be highly proficient. If they are not, patients can suffer, as the following case study describes.

## Case study: Switching off the life support by mistake

*Jamie had a car accident in 2002 that left him paralysed from the neck down (tetraplegic). It means he cannot breathe unless a machine (ventilator) is connected to his windpipe via a hole in his neck (tracheostomy). In spite of his high level of disability, Jamie was cared for at home. He was mentally alert, able to engage in meaningful discussions, used voice-activated computer technology to access the internet and write emails, and got about in a motorised wheelchair (if helped to get in and out). Jamie's main nursing need concerned his breathing as he was totally dependent on his ventilator machine. The NHS Trust entrusted his care to a private nursing agency. Jamie became worried about the quality of care he received and had a camera installed in January 2009 to video his care. It was done quite openly and there was a sign to inform nurses the camera was recording so that Jamie's family could check that he was all right.*

*Soon after the camera was installed, an agency nurse who had had no training or experience in the use of ventilator machines was attending to Jamie. The nurse found a switch that was turned on and decided to turn it off, an alarm sounded (warning not to turn ventilator machine off). Jamie could not speak without air so he frantically made a clicking noise with his tongue on the roof of his mouth (as he had been trained to do in an emergency) to show he was in distress. The nurse attempted to resuscitate him but wrongly placed a portable ventilation bag (Ambu® bag) over his mouth instead of the opening in his neck (the only way air could get to his lungs). Someone dialled 999, paramedics arrived, resuscitated Jamie and turned the ventilator machine back on. Jamie survived but suffered serious brain damage due to 20 minutes without oxygen. These events were captured by Jamie's camera, recorded onto his computer, and found by his sister. The nurse was suspended subject to an NMC investigation, and the NHS Trust instigated a review of policies with a view to preventing such tragedies from happening again in future.*

*(Adapted from BBC, 2010)*

Jamie's case study begs many questions about the organisation and delivery of care in the community such as: Why did the NHS Trust not have their own trained district nurses to oversee such specialist care? Why did the nursing agency delegate Jamie's care to a nurse who was not qualified to do so? Here we will focus on the nurse's own accountability for her decision-making and actions, as revealed by the video evidence. No criminal charges were brought against the nurse, which means the police believe it was accidental rather than a deliberate attempt to harm Jamie. There is no justification for switching off the ventilator machine, and we do not know why the nurse did so as no comment has been made pending the NMC investigation. Without Jamie's foresight in fitting a camera we would not have evidence of what happened. It highlights the point that we demonstrate our accountability for providing safe, competent nursing care each moment we are on duty. It is unusual for this to be observed and video recorded, but in a sense we need to imagine that this is happening all the time. If we stop to think 'Would I be happy for a video of how I just spoke to a patient or gave an injection to be seen by the NMC?', it would remind us not to do anything that we cannot justify being in the best interests of patients. In Activity 10.3 you are asked to explore various implications of the case study in more detail.

## Activity 10.3                         *Critical thinking*

The case study shows what can go wrong when nurses find themselves out of their depth and carry out tasks they are not competent to perform using medical devices unfamiliar to them. In this activity you are asked to reflect on how the nurse in the case study might have avoided endangering Jamie's life, permanently injuring him and increasing his already severe disability. You are then asked to relate this to your own practice. Please answer the following questions.

1. When the agency nurse discovered the severity of Jamie's disability and realised she did not have the knowledge or skills to care for him competently, what should she have done?
2. What may have stopped her from acknowledging she lacked competence to care for Jamie?
3. When the agency nurse noticed that a switch had been left on and was concerned about it, what alternative action should she have taken rather than turning it off?
4. What may have stopped her from deciding to take more appropriate alternative action?
5. If you are asked to perform a procedure you do not feel competent in, what would you do?
6. If you find a switch on an unfamiliar medical device left switched on, what would you do?

*Some possible answers can be found at the end of the chapter.*

Activity 10.3 and Jamie's case study underline how important it is for nurses to know what they are doing, and not do what they are not competent to perform. In order to be accountable we have to justify our decision-making. We can only justify decision-making if we understand how our actions are of benefit to patients, including reference to relevant supporting evidence. We may also be able to justify a decision not to perform a procedure where we can argue we lack the skills to do so safely and effectively. This would not excuse us from ensuring the patient is attended to by someone who has the required level of clinical competence. So far we have looked at how observations of our practice can be used in holding us to account for decision-making. We will now look at how written records of care can also be used for this purpose.

# Accountability and written records of our practice

Just as we need to base decision-making and nursing activities on relevant research evidence, current policies and clinical guidelines, we are also required to keep up-to-date written records as evidence of the care we have given. Various functions of good record keeping are listed in *Record keeping: Guidance for nurses and midwives* (NMC, 2009b, p2), including the following.

- Helping to improve accountability.
- Showing how decisions related to patient care were made.
- Supporting effective clinical judgements and decisions.
- Making continuity of care easier.

- Providing documentary evidence of services delivered.
- Promoting better communication and sharing of information between members of the multi-professional healthcare team.
- Helping to identify risks, and enabling early detection of complications.
- Supporting clinical audit, research, allocation of resources and performance planning.
- Helping to address complaints or legal processes.

Handwritten or electronic notes, reflective journals, observation charts, drug charts, care plans and assessment forms contribute to an audit trail of decision-making that we can be asked to explain, justify and defend. In the next case study a newly qualified nurse shows how problems can occur when record keeping is inaccurate or not kept up to date in administering medicines.

## Case study: Signing the drug chart

*Tracy registered as a nurse six months ago and has recently completed additional training in administering intravenous fluids and medication. Robert is due to receive a powerful intravenous antibiotic, and Tracy checks the drug with another nurse before attending to him. After giving the antibiotic Robert's bedside telephone rings and he asks Tracy if she'd mind telling whoever it is that he is having treatment and not 'up to talking' at the moment. Tracy obliges, puts the phone down, and leaves Robert to rest, completely forgetting to sign that he had the antibiotic on the drug chart. When the next shift takes over they give Robert an extra dose because there is no record of him having had the antibiotic earlier. When the mistake is discovered a clinical incident form is filled in. Matron asks Tracy to apologise to Robert and to inform his consultant about it, which she does. She feels terribly embarrassed and vows not to be so easily distracted from finishing what she is doing, and to make sure she remembers to sign the drug chart in future. Robert did not suffer any ill effects but Tracy felt it was more by luck than judgement on her part.*

The case study highlights how important accurate record keeping is in documenting patient care and the potential problems of not doing so. It also reinforces the point that nurses are not only accountable for what they do but also for what they do not do (not signing drug chart). As quoted in the introduction, we are *personally accountable for actions and omissions* (NMC, 2008, p1).

If Robert's bedside phone had not rung, then Tracy would not have been distracted from signing the chart. As nurses we cannot simply hope that nothing distracts us from carrying out procedures because there will always be 'a phone call' or some other demand on our attention, so we have to find better ways of dealing with them. Activity 10.4 asks you to explore Tracy's accountability for her decision-making in more detail.

## Activity 10.4                                                   *Decision-making*

Decision-making involves selecting a course of action from the available alternatives. In this activity you are asked to evaluate Tracy's decision-making, consider what else she might have done, and what can be learnt from such mistakes. Please answer the following questions.

*continued overleaf . . .*

*continued . . .*

1. Do you think Tracy was justified in not signing the drug chart? If yes, why? If not, why not?
2. Do you think Tracy was justified in answering the phone? If yes, why? If not, why not?
3. What alternative options were available to Tracy when Robert's bedside phone rang?
4. Do you think the matron was justified in asking Tracy to apologise to Robert and inform the consultant about the mistake that had been made? If yes, why? If not, why not?
5. Look at the NMC functions of good record keeping (above) and select three that were undermined by Tracy's actions. How would signing a drug chart address these points?
6. Given that Robert did not appear to suffer any ill effects from Tracy's oversight, why do you think it is important that she learns not to make the same mistake again?

*Some possible answers can be found at the end of the chapter.*

Activity 10.4 and the related case study highlight the fine line between nurses helping as opposed to harming patients (beneficence versus non-maleficence, Chapter 9). Tracy's caring instinct was to do what Robert wanted by answering the phone for him, but this incident taught her to think more carefully about the pros and cons of doing so. By allowing herself to be distracted from completing the intravenous procedure properly rather than helping Robert, she exposed him to possible danger. In being held to account for her mistake Tracy was made acutely aware that being a caring person is not enough to be an effective nurse. We also need to be vigilant in continually assessing risks associated with our decision-making and related actions, and then minimise and control such risks to avoid endangering patients. This is easier said than done, but it is vital that we do so.

As the healthcare professionals having most contact with patients, we have more decision-making opportunities in assessing and addressing their needs and preferences than others. In other words, we are accountable for a great many nursing decisions every day. It is why observations of our practice by patients and others, and written records of what we have done are key sources of evidence in holding us to account for our decision-making. Through clinical governance this is happening all the time at a local level, as shown in the case study. In a sense Tracy was held to account for confusing kindness with her duty of care to competently complete the intravenous procedure and sign the drug chart. By deviating from standardised procedure (Chapter 5) Tracy exposed Robert to greater risk, and left herself open to criticism. It is fortunate the outcome of her mistake did not adversely affect Robert's health and well-being. Knowing that the outcome could have been worse emphasises the importance of learning from and avoiding such mistakes in future. Being accountable goes hand in hand with striving to improve on the care we give to patients. We also saw in Jamie's case study that nurses may be required to account for decision-making at a national level if the outcomes of mistakes are more serious or professional conduct is called into question. This leads us to look at how the NMC Code reminds us of our accountability in all types of decision-making.

# Accountability in all types of decision-making

Accountability has been identified in this book as a decision-making theme in its own right because knowing that we are answerable for our decisions as nurses affects how we make them. However, in itself, accountability does not tell us how to make a decision, only that it should be justifiable as being in the best interests of patients. In practice, all of the types of decision-making discussed in this book need to be combined with accountability because without it there is no way of confirming that we have 'practised what we preach'.

Table 10.2 shows how we can apply relevant extracts from the Code (NMC, 2008) regarding our professional accountability as nurses to each of the other decision-making types discussed in this book. If we apply it to Robert's case study, we see that there is a clash between collaborative and standardised decision-making as Tracy (the nurse) interrupted the intravenous procedure to respond to Robert's request that she answers his phone. If we apply Table 10.2 to Jamie's case study, it would appear that the nurse did not demonstrate her accountability regarding any of the identified decision-making types or related extracts of the NMC Code of professional conduct.

| Decision making | Relevant extracts from NMC Code (2008) re accountability |
|---|---|
| *Collaborative* | *You must recognise and respect the contribution that people make to their own care and wellbeing* (p3); and *You must work cooperatively within teams and respect the skills, expertise and contributions of your colleagues* (p5). |
| *Observation* | *You must complete and keep clear and accurate records of the discussions you have, the assessments you make, the treatment and medicines you give and how effective these have been* (p8). |
| *Systematic* | *You must work with colleagues to monitor the quality of your work and maintain the safety of those in your care* (p5). |
| *Standardised* | *You must deliver care based on the best available evidence or best practice* (p7). |
| *Prioritising* | *You must report your concerns in writing if problems in the environment of care are putting people at risk* (p6). |
| *Experience and intuition* | *You must have the knowledge and skills for safe and effective practice when working without direct supervision* (p7). |
| *Reflective* | *You must take part in appropriate learning and practice activities that maintain and develop your competence and performance* (p7). |
| *Ethical sensitivity* | *You must respect and support people's rights to accept or decline treatment and care* (p4). |
| *Confidence* | *You must uphold the reputation of your profession at all times* (p10). |

*Table 10.2: Nurses' professional accountability in all types of decision-making*

It may seem ironic that as nurses aspire to more professional autonomy they encounter more accountability for their decision-making and nursing interventions. This is an in-built safeguard to protect patients as the power to make vital decisions regarding people's lives is tempered by the requirement that such decisions be open to scrutiny by others. This leads us on to clarifying why it is that accountability for nursing decisions is so important.

# Why is accountability important?

So far we have established that accountability means having to account for (explain and justify) our decisions to patients, public, employers and the nursing profession, who observe our practice and may scrutinise written records of the care we have provided. At this point we need to be clear about the purpose of professional accountability in nursing. According to Griffith and Tengnah (2010) accountability has four functions – *protective*, *deterrent*, *regulatory* and *educative*. We will now explore what this means by relating functions to accountability for nursing decisions.

## Protective function

This is the primary aim of professional accountability for nursing decisions. As we saw in Chapter 9, our first duty as nurses is not to harm patients (non-maleficence) by our actions or lack of action. Potential benefits of patient care are easily undermined by unprofessional behaviour and by errors. An example is the case of the premature baby described in Chapter 9, who weighed less than two pounds at birth and was helped to survive until at four months he died after nurses put too much sodium chloride in his intravenous infusion. The NMC is responsible for protecting the public by investigating complaints about nurses' fitness to practise and, if necessary, instigate sanctions. Sanctions include: i) a caution not to repeat behaviour; ii) making a condition of practice (e.g. requiring nurse to have more training or supervision in order to continue practising); iii) suspension pending further investigations; and iv) a striking off order (nurse removed from the professional register).

In 2009–2010, 2,988 allegations questioning nurses' fitness to practise were made. This is 0.4 per cent of the total number of registered nurses (662,283) at the time. The allegations were made by employers (40 per cent), public (22 per cent), police (19 per cent), other professionals (2 per cent), and others (17 per cent). The allegations include lack of competence and more serious professional misconduct, as follows:

> *Dishonesty, patient abuse, lack of competence, failure to maintain adequate records, incorrect administration of drugs, neglect of basic care, unsafe clinical practice, failure to collaborate with colleagues, colleague abuse, failure to report incidents, failure to act in an emergency, accessing illegal pornography, and violence.*

The NMC Conduct and Competence Committee instigated sanctions in 925 of these cases, of which 202 were striking off orders (see NMC website link at the end of this chapter for more information). This might seem small comfort for patients who suffered from poor care or abuse. They or their families may be entitled to claim compensation from NHS Trusts and nurses in recognition that their health and well-being were not protected as they should have been, when negligent care and unjustifiable and indefensible decision-making is evident.

# Deterrent function

Of course, the best type of protection is to prevent mistakes in healthcare from occurring in the first place. The knowledge that we are always being observed, our performance evaluated and records of decision-making and care delivery audited reminds us to always act professionally. Hearing about nurses being suspended or dismissed from their jobs, or found unfit for practice and struck off the NMC register due to professional misconduct underlines how we are accountable to a higher authority that has the power to take away our livelihood. This discourages us from emulating unprofessional behaviour that undermines the public's trust and confidence in nurses. For example, one of the nurses involved in administering a fatal amount of sodium chloride to the young baby referred to above was not only investigated by the NMC regarding her role in this, she was also sacked by the NHS Trust for gross misconduct. She had uploaded onto her social networking site photos of herself asleep next to (and supposedly looking after) the baby who later died. Imagine how the parents of the baby boy would have felt about this. By sacking the nurse, her employers clearly showed that such behaviour is unacceptable and will not be tolerated. It is also a 'wake-up call' for other nurses to keep their professional and personal lives separate in relation to social networking sites. The deterrent function of accountability therefore gives us professional boundaries that it is foolish to cross.

# Regulatory function

Whereas the deterrent function dissuades us from doing what we should not do, the regulatory function of accountability guides us in what we should do to justify public trust in nurses. The Code for nurses and midwives begins *The people in your care must be able to trust you with their health and well-being* (NMC, 2008, p1) and then lists standards of professional conduct that enable patients to trust us to help them. This is the regulatory framework defining who we are as nurses, and by complying with it we demonstrate our professional accountability. It is very important because if we adhere to the Code in our clinical practice we increase the chances that our decision-making and nursing actions will benefit rather than harm patients. Complying with the Code does not guarantee that complications will not occur, but if they do, we are able to show that we did what we could to achieve the best possible outcome for patients. In this way abiding by the Code not only protects patients, it also protects our reputation as nurses.

Other regulatory frameworks we have to abide by include the NHS Constitution (discussed earlier) specifying principles and values all parties need to respect throughout the NHS. NICE or other evidence-based clinical guidelines underpinning standardised decision-making (Chapter 5) in numerous clinical procedures represent a practical regulatory framework for everyday use. Many regulatory frameworks influencing our clinical practice have a legal basis – see Table 10.3.

Table 10.3 gives an indication of many legally enforceable regulatory frameworks that impact on our role and duties as nurses. It may seem a lot for us to take in, but in practice the policies and procedures in clinical areas incorporate relevant aspects of this myriad of legislation. The more we delve into accountability, the more there is to learn, and we will look into this a bit more now.

| Relevant Act or Order | Examples of application in nursing |
|---|---|
| Equality Act 2010 | No discrimination regarding age, sex, race or disability |
| Health Act 2009 | Apply principles and values of the NHS Constitution |
| Health and Social Care Act 2008 | Cooperate with Care Quality Commission inquiries |
| Mental Health Act 2007 (and 1983) | Voluntary or compulsory criteria to treat mental disorder |
| Nursing and Midwifery Order 2001 | Comply with NMC Code of professional, ethical conduct |
| Freedom of Information Act 2000 | Patients' right of access to view records of their care |
| Data Protection Act 1998 | Only authorised access to patients' confidential data |
| Human Rights Act 1998 | Respect patients' right to life and to dignified treatment |
| Children Act 1989 | Duty to report suspected non-accidental injury of a child |
| Health and Safety at Work Act 1974 | Obligation to report safety concerns within clinical areas |
| Misuse of Drugs Act 1971 | Safely store, record, give (if prescribed) controlled drugs |

*Table 10.3: Examples of legally enforceable regulatory frameworks*

# Educative function

Accountability requires us to explain, justify and defend our actions to others, and we cannot do this unless we think about and articulate reasons and evidence supporting our decision-making. Hence, the very act of demonstrating our accountability is potentially educational, prompting us to be aware of what we are doing and why, risks associated with our actions, how competent we feel in managing these, and whether we have given anyone cause to make a complaint. Simon, a newly qualified nurse, identified three questions to sum up his understanding of accountability: 'What happens if it goes wrong? What can happen to the patient? What can happen to me?' In the next case study, Sean, another newly qualified nurse, described a situation he found quite challenging in deciding whether or not to give a patient prescribed discretionary medication.

## Case study: PRN medication

*Sean's first staff nurse job is in an acute mental health unit where Nick, aged 26, is being treated for anxiety and depression. Along with his regular medication Nick is prescribed an extra dose of anti-anxiety PRN medication. PRN is short for* pro re nata *(Latin), meaning to be taken when required. Sean had to use his discretion in judging whether it was appropriate to give the additional medication, given that it could be addictive and Nick had a history of drug abuse. 'I noticed Nick was making a habit of coming everyday for the PRN medication and I wondered whether he really needed it, or was misusing it. It was almost as if he treated it as an additional regular supply but that was not what it was intended for. Many times I did not feel he looked particularly agitated to warrant the PRN dose. Then I thought he might feel agitated but not show visible signs, and the PRN was prescribed so maybe I should give it to him when he asks. I decided to ask Nick what he was agitated about and a couple of times he just started smiling, so I didn't give him the PRN on those days. There were other days when he could give a valid reason why he was feeling stressed, and so I felt more confident giving it then. It was something I reviewed all the time to try to ensure the PRN medication was used for therapeutic reasons.'*

The case study shows how Sean applied accountability in nursing decisions. He could have simply given the PRN medication every time Nick asked but he felt this was unjustifiable when the evidence suggested additional medication was not actually required. Using Simon's questions (page 170) as a guide, we can review Sean's decision-making further.

- What happens if it goes wrong? If Sean got it wrong, he would either give the PRN medication when Nick did not really need it or not give it when he did.
- What happens to the patient? Nick would either be over- or under-medicated, neither of which would be therapeutic.
- What happens to me? Sean would either be colluding with drug misuse by Nick or upsetting Nick by not trusting him when he was genuinely in need of PRN anti-anxiety medication.

There are many ways we can explain, justify and defend our actions, and Table 10.4 relates Sean's accountability for decision-making to conceptions of nursing.

| Conceptions of nursing | Accountability in decision-making |
|---|---|
| Caring | Ensuring PRN medication is beneficial and not harmful to Nick |
| Listening and being there | Give Nick time to explain what might be worrying him |
| Practical procedures | Safely giving or not giving PRN medication, as appropriate |

*— continued overleaf . . .*

*Table 10.4: Integrating conceptions of nursing and accountability in decision-making*

| Conceptions of nursing | Accountability in decision-making |
|---|---|
| Knowledge and understanding | Anti-anxiety drugs, doses, side-effects, uses and abuses |
| Communicating | Asking Nick directly what he is feeling agitated about |
| Patience | Control possible sense of irritation that Nick is 'trying it on' |
| Teamwork | Entrusted by doctor to decide if PRN medication is needed |
| Paperwork and electronic record | Recording medication given, and the interactions with Nick |
| Empathising and non-judgemental | Appreciate that Nick may genuinely need PRN medication |
| Professional | Maintaining good relationship without colluding with Nick |

*Table 10.4: Continued*

Table 10.4 provides another example of how accountability for nursing decisions might be explained with reference to the ten conceptions of nursing. Matching accountability to each of the conceptions of nursing requires reflective learning, which contributes to its educative function. In Activity 10.5 you are asked to apply this to your own practice placement experience.

---

**Activity 10.5**                                                  *Reflection*

Although, as a student, you are not fully accountable for patient care, you are accountable for making good use of your learning opportunities in practice placements. With this in mind, identify an example when you were working with a patient and felt you made a meaningful contribution to their care. Then adapt Table 10.4 to map your example against the ten conceptions of nursing, indicating how justifiable your actions were in the same way that we did for Sean. It should help you to integrate an awareness of accountability with development as a nurse.

*As this activity is for your own private reflection, there is no outline answer included.*

---

## Chapter summary

This chapter discussed the nature of accountability for nursing decisions and how this requires us to be able to explain, justify and defend our decision-making. We noted that compliance with the NMC Code of conduct facilitates our professional accountability and that we also have to adhere to the principles and values of the NHS Constitution. We identified that we are primarily accountable to service users but also to employers, the NMC, and the law for our decision-making, actions and omissions. We looked at how we need to demonstrate accountability in everything we do as we are being constantly observed by patients, colleagues and others. Written records of the care we give also provide evidence of our decision-making, and whether it appears justified. We established that accountability is married to each of the other decision-making types discussed in this book and this was supported with reference to the NMC's code. We examined why accountability is so important in protecting patients and the wider public by ensuring that nurses deemed unfit for practice forfeit the right to do so. It was argued that this can help deter nurses from making the same mistakes. We looked at how a range of legally enforceable frameworks – not just the NMC Code – regulate our decision-making and conduct. It was argued that being continually aware of our accountability for decision-making is educational in its own right as it prompts us to question our practice and examine the strength of supporting evidence. Topical case studies and related activities highlighted the challenges faced by nurses, what happens if things go wrong, and how to effectively apply accountability in decision-making.

## Activities: brief outline answers

### Activity 10.1 Leadership and management (page 159)

You may have included the following points:

1. Reggie's possible justification for whistling:
   Boost morale, de-stress, relax, convey happiness at work.
   Was not in direct contact with patients during the activity.
   Unaware he was causing a distraction or disturbance.

2. Ward manager's possible justification to stop Reggie whistling:
   Distracting her while talking to relative.
   Relative could also have been distracted.
   It might be viewed as unprofessional behaviour in an acute medical setting.
   It could possibly disturb patients who need to rest.
   Reggie may not hear if a patient or colleague needs assistance.
   Disposal of used needles/syringes part of infection control to be taken seriously.

## Activity 10.3 Critical thinking (page 164)

You may have included the following points.

1.  Phone nursing agency, talk to the duty manager, explain she was not able to care for Jamie safely or effectively as his needs were beyond her experience and training, and ask for a suitable replacement. Explain to Jamie reason for the delay in attending to his care needs. Request further training and supervision from agency before being asked to care for Jamie.
2.  Fear that she might lose her job with nursing agency; too proud to admit ignorance; lack of critical awareness of risks posed to Jamie in attempting to care for him when she did not understand what she was doing; unfamiliarity with professional code of conduct in nursing – *You must recognise and work within the limitations of your competence* (NMC, 2008, p7).
3.  Leave the switch alone as she did not know what it was for and at that time Jamie was not in any distress so there was no reason to think leaving it switched on would harm him. Up until the time the nurse turned off ventilator machine Jamie could speak so if she was unsure about anything she could have asked him, and he would have explained things to her.
4.  She may have felt a compulsion 'to be seen to be doing something' not realising she was putting Jamie in grave danger. She may have underestimated Jamie's lucid mind (due to his physical disability) and not realised he was an expert in his own care who could advise her. Perhaps she didn't like being videoed and thought she was turning the camera off.
5.  Admit you have not done it before or not reached a competent standard; request you observe a competent nurse performing the procedure before you attempt it; read up on the procedure – its purpose, equipment needed and technique; familiarise yourself with the patient concerned and how the procedure is intended to be of benefit regarding their medical condition; only then agree to perform the procedure under the watchful eye of a suitably experienced nurse.
6.  If you do not know what it is for, leave it turned on, check whether the medical device or piece of equipment is connected to a patient and if that patient appears distressed, report this to a senior nursing colleague straightaway, find out what the medical device is for and any observations you need to make regarding its use.

## Activity 10.4 Decision-making (pages 165–6)

You may have included the following points.

1.  There were mitigating circumstances (first time doing activity, phone interruption), Tracy's intentions were good, and Robert did not suffer any ill effects. However, not signing a drug chart cannot be justified as it was her duty and not doing so exposed Robert to higher risk.
2.  Tracy answered the phone because Robert asked, so she was attentive and accountable to his preferences. However, it was only justifiable if it did not disrupt the intravenous procedure and we know that it did because she forgot to sign the drug chart.
3.  Tracy's possible alternative options: ignore the phone ringing; tell Robert she is sorry but cannot answer it as she needs to finish the procedure (sign chart, dispose of syringe etc.); tell Robert she will answer the phone when she has signed the chart, cleared away and washed hands; if phone is bothering Robert, suggest he tells the caller to ring back later, or unplug the phone.
4.  Matron was justified because it is better to admit mistakes than cover them up; Robert was entitled to know what happened and to get an apology; the medical team also needed to be informed to take any necessary action; it reinforced Tracy's sense of accountability for her actions/omissions; and it facilitated her learning from experience not to repeat the mistake.
5.  Three points from functions of good record keeping that were undermined, for example: i) *Making continuity of care easier* – if the drug chart had been signed, the next shift would not have made the mistake of repeating the dose; ii) *Providing documentary evidence of services delivered* – if the drug chart had been signed, it would have been evident that the intravenous antibiotic had been given; iii) *Promoting better*

*communication and sharing of information between members of the multi-professional healthcare team* – if the drug chart was unsigned, the next shift would not know whether or not the drug had been given.

6.  It is important that Tracy learns not to make such mistakes because they expose patients to unnecessary risks. She felt it was more by luck than judgement on her part that the outcome was not more serious; other patients might have had a more serious reaction than Robert, and other drugs may be more dangerous if double the prescribed dose is wrongly given.

## Further reading

**Griffith, R and Tengnah, C** (2010) *Law and Professional Issues in Nursing*, 2nd edition. Exeter: Learning Matters.

Chapter 2 provides a comprehensive overview of accountability in nursing practice.

## Useful websites

**www.nmc-uk.org/About-us/Statistics/Statistics-about-fitness-to-practise-hearings/**

NMC website that has annual reports from 2000 to 2010 with details of all allegations, investigations and sanctions.

# Chapter 11
# Confidence in clinical decision-making

> **Chapter aims**
>
> By the end of this chapter, you should be able to:
>
> - explain what confidence in decision-making means;
> - relate confidence to your 'three categories of selves';
> - identify what develops or inhibits nurses' confidence;
> - apply confidence in all types of decision-making;
> - plan how to develop confidence as a registered nurse.

# Introduction

In this final chapter of our journey, we round things off by exploring the nature and function of **confidence** in clinical judgement and decision-making. The NMC emphasises its importance in enabling nurses to be self-directing (autonomous), co-operative and effective healthcare team members. We also need to gain the trust of and inspire confidence in those we care for and work with (see Essential Skills Clusters box). If we are not self-directing, we will find it difficult to make our own decisions. If we have problems working as part of a team, we will be less effective in contributing to patients' integrated care pathways. If we cannot get patients to trust us, they will lack confidence in our ability to help them, and feel anxious about their health and well-being. Hence, confidence is a vital ingredient nurses need to incorporate in clinical decision-making.

We start by clarifying what confidence in clinical decision-making means. We explore Reinharz's (1997) 'three categories of selves' in relation to our personal (self) and professional (theoretical and practical) confidence. We then look at what develops or inhibits confidence in decision-making and explore how confidence is applied within other decision-making types discussed in this book. Ways of continuing to develop confidence in clinical decision-making after qualifying as a registered nurse are briefly outlined. As in previous chapters, case studies and activities are used to engage your interest and assist you in integrating theory and practice.

# What is confidence in clinical decision-making?

There are a number of meanings associated with the term 'confidence', as shown below.

*1. Trust or belief in a person or thing.*

*2. Faith in one's own ability; self-assurance.*

*3. A secret confided to someone.*

*4. A relationship of mutual trust.*

(Chambers, 2010)

All of these meanings are relevant and applied within confidence in clinical decision-making, but they require further clarification and qualification. We want patients, relatives, team members and others to trust us to help them (through safe and effective clinical judgement and decision-making as discussed in this book), but in doing so we are morally obliged not to abuse that trust. Confidence tricksters are skilled in soliciting people's trust in order to cheat or harm them in some way, so trusting people and being trusted by others is not necessarily always a good thing. If nurses abuse their privileged position, for example, by stealing from, abusing or sexually assaulting patients, they risk criminal prosecution, being sacked, and being struck off the NMC register (see Chapter 9). We also have to be aware that some medical conditions, such as toxic confusional states, head injuries, mental disorders and drug dependency, can make it difficult to trust the accuracy of what patients are telling us, without carefully checking other sources of evidence.

In other words, developing a trusting relationship is complex – not something we can confirm by ticking a box – and we have to continually work at developing and maintaining trust with patients. As well as trusting others and getting others to trust us, we need to trust in our own abilities. It is necessary to be self-assured in order to have the 'courage of our convictions' and do what we believe to be the right thing. The following case study describes how a new nursing student's lack of self-confidence constrains her ability to make quite basic decisions.

## Case study: Ask mum

*Amy, aged 18, had recently commenced a nursing preparation programme. She was asked what she understood by decision-making, and what experience she had of it. Amy did not know how to answer the question, so she was asked how she would go about planning a shopping trip. This is what she replied: 'I talk to my mum about everything. If she agrees with it, I will go and do it; if she doesn't, then I rethink it. She doesn't like certain colours on me so I would have to get something that she liked. In fact, she always comes along to do clothes shopping with me.'*

The case study suggests that Amy is compliant and totally dependent on her mother, who makes quite basic decisions on her behalf and overrides any expressed preferences. It highlights how our self-confidence as nurses is helped or hindered by previous life experience (or lack of it). It may seem a little worrying to think that patients are entrusting their health and well-being to someone who might say to them, 'Wait a minute, I've got to ask mum.' On the other hand, it may be easier for someone like Amy to increase their self-confidence (as we shall see later) than it is for an over-confident person to rein it in to a more appropriate level. An over-confident student may be over-compensating for a lack of confidence, and it is difficult for them to acknowledge this. It means that they pose more of a risk to patients (by undertaking activities they are not competent to perform safely) than a student who always seeks guidance. Activity 11.1 asks you to imagine that you have to supervise an over-confident nursing student.

---

**Activity 11.1**                                    *Leadership and management*

Imagine you have completed your nursing programme and are awaiting confirmation of your NMC registration. You are working in a clinical area where you have worked for the last three months, and one of two qualified nurses on your shift has reported sick. When the remaining staff nurse has a break you are left in charge of a group of patients with Nathan, a second-year nursing student, to help you. After answering a phone call at the nurses' station you notice three patients (suffering from diabetes, epilepsy and dementia) and the nursing students are missing. One of the remaining patients tells you they have just left the unit. You go to the door, see them in the corridor and ask Nathan what he thinks he is doing. He replies, 'Chill out! We're just off to the hospital shop for a bit of "retail therapy" to relieve the boredom, and give these guys a bit of exercise.' What would you do to ensure the safety of all the patients you are responsible for? What would you say to Nathan in order for him to understand the inappropriateness of his actions?

*Some possible answers can be found at the end of the chapter.*

---

The case study and Activity 11.1 highlight the need to get the balance right between under- and over-confidence. A self-assured nurse is someone patients can trust to help them rather than expose them to unnecessary, potentially high-risk situations, due to misguided decision-making. Activity 11.1 also shows how self-assurance is needed if one is to be an assertive advocate on behalf of patients when a colleague or anyone else appears to be jeopardising their health and safety. Understanding that some patients are more vulnerable than others requires knowing them as individuals, their health problems, medical conditions and personal circumstances. It requires confidence in our knowledge of evidence-based practice and its effective application. This is where we have to combine personal (self) and professional (theoretical and practical) assurance to inspire patients to trust our decision-making in delivering safe, high-quality nursing care. So, for the purposes of this chapter, confidence in decision-making is understood to mean:

> *self-assurance from previous experience or achievements and professional assurance (respecting confidentiality, applying evidence-based practice) to inspire patients to trust you to help them, and enable you to explain, justify and defend your decisions.*

# Three categories of selves in personal and professional confidence

When we speak of self-confidence, self-assurance or self-awareness, it suggests we have just one 'self'. Reinharz (1997) argues we have many 'selves' and that understanding different ways they influence our perceptions, beliefs, attitudes and judgement is important. She is not saying that we all have multiple 'Jekyll and Hyde' personalities. Rather, she is saying we have many contrasting strands of thoughts, feelings and experiences woven together, shaping who we are. Often we are not aware of them or the different ways that they can influence our judgement. Reinharz was concerned that unless researchers have a better psychological understanding of themselves, personal biases and mistaken beliefs remain unchecked. This can result in their misinterpretation of the behaviour they are researching, and inaccurate reporting of evidence.

Like researchers, nurses interact with people to find out information that informs future action, so it is equally important for us to be confident in the accuracy of our observations. Applying reflexivity (Chapter 8) can help us to monitor and control our potential biases, which could otherwise distort our understanding of what we think is true. Reinharz identified three categories of selves that can be used to enhance our critical thinking, reflection and reflexivity in this respect.

1. *Brought selves* – past experience shapes our understanding.
2. *Research-based selves* – scientific evidence shapes our understanding.
3. *Situationally created selves* – interacting with others shapes our understanding.

There are many different strands within each of the three categories, which is why they are referred to as 'selves' rather than 'self'. For example: past experience includes happiness and sadness, successes and failures; there are many different types and ways of obtaining evidence; and we interact with various people and social contexts at different (and unique) moments in time. Table 11.1 cross-references Reinharz's selves to nurses' personal and professional confidence.

| Three categories of selves | Personal confidence | Professional confidence |
|---|---|---|
| 'Brought selves' (PERSONAL) | Personality, life history influences: how we perceive self and others; how accurate or biased our view of the world is; unresolved emotional 'baggage'; past successes and failures; how self-confident we feel meeting people for the first time or dealing with a new challenge | |
| 'Research-based selves' (THEORETICAL) | | University input influences: accessing relevant information; development of critical thinking to evaluate research evidence; understanding health problems |

*Table 11.1: Nurses' personal and professional confidence – three categories of selves*

| Three categories of selves | Personal confidence | Professional confidence |
|---|---|---|
| | | and treatment methods; nurses' role in decision-making; reflection in lifelong learning; confidence to articulate views |
| 'Situationally created selves' (PRACTICAL) | | Work-based learning in clinical practice influences: nurses' identity; engaging with patients, team members; apply theory to practice; develop clinical decision-making skills; respect patients' confidentiality; develop confidence from sense of achievement helping patients |

*Table 11.1: Continued*

Table 11.1 shows how Reinharz's three categories of selves can be used to map and assess how confident we feel as nurses, personally and professionally, in our decision-making. Cross-referencing our personal assumptions with theoretical evidence or practical experience can also challenge potential biases we may bring with us from the past, as the next case study reveals.

## Case study: I imagined doctors would be arrogant

*Graham is about to complete his nursing programme, mental health pathway. When asked how he perceives nursing now compared to when he began, he said, 'I imagined before I started the programme that the doctors would be quite arrogant, if you like, and difficult, but I found the opposite actually. I found them to be genuinely quite friendly. They came straightaway if we needed them to review a patient, were always interested in discussing diagnoses, treatments and legal issues with us, and gave me useful information and advice about cognitive therapy for my case study.'*

The case study shows that our past experience (brought selves) can give rise to biased opinion and attitudes that might be resistant to change. Fortunately, Graham's prejudice was not so fixed, and when he found it was not supported by his clinical experience ('situationally created selves') and that the opposite seemed to be true (doctors he met were friendly, not arrogant), he revised his judgement accordingly. Applying Reinharz's three categories of selves, therefore, increases our reflexivity by checking out assumptions against alternative types and strength of evidence.

Table 11.1 also reinforces how nursing combines both personal and professional (theoretical and practical) development. The personal dimension may not receive as much attention as the other two either at university or in practice settings, but without it how can we feel confident in our decision-making? Theory, research and practical nursing skills that we learn also add to our repertoire of personal experience (brought selves), which influences how self-confident we feel for our next clinical encounter. Ultimately, clinical decision-making and nursing actions do affect the *personal* worlds of our patients, so not losing sight of our own personal needs can help remind us to be more sensitive and responsive to patients' personal preferences. This can be easily overlooked as we develop our 'research-based selves' amid the complexity and technology of twenty-first-century evidence-based nursing. However, good communication skills and caring qualities are what patients value the most about nurses, so it is important for us to integrate and apply personal, theoretical and practical aspects in patient-centred care. Table 11.1 shows this can be facilitated by applying Reinharz's three categories of selves (brought, research-based and situationally created) to develop personal and professional confidence in decision-making. Activity 11.2 asks you to use the three categories of selves to assess your own confidence.

## Activity 11.2                                                    *Reflection*

Read through what has been written above concerning Reinharz's three categories of selves and personal–professional confidence in decision-making. Look at how Table 11.1 describes the relationships between them and then answer the following.

1. Look at the description of personal confidence in relation to brought selves (Table 11.1) and rate your own level of confidence in this respect on a scale of 1–10.
2. Look at professional (theoretical) confidence in relation to research-based selves (Table 11.1) and rate your own level of confidence in this respect on a scale of 1–10.
3. Look at professional (practical) confidence in relation to situationally created selves (Table 11.1) and rate your own level of confidence in this respect on a scale of 1–10.
4. Which of the above areas do you feel most confident in?
5. How much variation is there in your confidence scores?
6. Which of the above areas do you feel least confident in?
7. What do you feel would help you to increase your confidence?
8. How are you planning to develop your confidence in this area?

*As this is for your own reflection and professional development, there is no outline answer given, but you may find it helpful to discuss a possible action plan with someone that you trust.*

Activity 11.2 invited you to explore and assess your own levels of personal, theoretical and practical confidence in clinical judgement and decision-making, by applying Reinharz's three categories of selves. By honestly self-assessing areas we lack confidence in we give ourselves an opportunity to do something about it that can benefit us both personally and professionally. We now turn to look at what inhibits and what develops confidence in clinical decision-making.

# What inhibits and what develops confidence in clinical decision-making?

In this section we look at personal, theoretical and practical factors that can enable us to gain or lose confidence in our decision-making ability as nurses. Table 11.2 uses extracts from research into nursing students' clinical decision-making (Standing, 2005) for this purpose.

| Factors | Inhibiting confidence | Developing confidence |
|---|---|---|
| Personal (brought selves) | • lack of relevant experience e.g. *lady had miscarriage, I didn't know what to say, I just felt inadequate*<br>• bullied and victimised in past<br>• bereavement, relationship breakdown, and ill health | • relevant past experience<br>• advice and encouragement e.g. *manager felt I was ready for nurse training, I thought yes I'm going for it*<br>• stable supportive personal relationships, and 'growing up' |
| Theoretical (research-based selves) | • not enough sessions in skills lab plus relevance of lectures to nursing practice not always clear<br>• theory-practice gap e.g. *theory is patient-centred care – but in practice it is often task-orientated*<br>• after qualifying less time to read | • presenting seminar to group e.g. *everyone picks apart what you say, I was nervous but grew very confident*<br>• teach other students procedures<br>• keep up-to-date with journals e.g. *I read journals, surprised how much I knew already, I felt more confident* |
| Practical (situationally created selves) | • not enough nurses on duty, and shortage of the right equipment<br>• stress of meeting health targets<br>• death of patient you cared for<br>• lack of clinical supervision<br>• making mistakes e.g. *patient did not come to harm but could have, I still get upset about it* | • using decision-making skills e.g. *you come out of your shell, by being in a situation you learn to deal with it*<br>• mentors instil confidence e.g. *mentor said 'tell me what to do' – scary but it made me think how to plan care*<br>• being trusted as a team member<br>• delegated responsibilities e.g. *nominated as case conference speaker* |

*Table 11.2: Factors that inhibit or develop confidence in clinical decision-making*

Table 11.2 suggests that confidence in clinical decision-making is a balancing act between inhibiting and developmental factors, including personal, theoretical and practical, or a combination thereof. Nurses are not robots; we are people, too. At any time stressful life events such as the death of a loved one can occur, and when this happens it can shake our confidence not just in our private life but also at work. Of course, we all react to stress in different ways and some of us might find it therapeutic to immerse ourselves in work to avoid having to think about such events. We also experience stress at work if clinical demand exceeds the capacity of healthcare providers to deal with it safely and effectively. Perceived stress is exacerbated if we make a mistake or a patient we know dies. At such times *we* may need taking care of a bit more, and mentoring or clinical supervision is useful in this respect, if it is available. As students, stress associated with theoretical factors is usually related to passing written assessments. As far as decision-making is concerned, theoretical factors can help to inform evidence-based decisions and explain them. If relevant theory has 'gone over our head' for one reason or another, we are disadvantaged in this respect. We may also have difficulty managing time in order to keep up to date, especially after we have qualified. If this happens, our evidence-based decision-making is 'past its sell-by date'. Activity 11.3 now asks you to relate Table 11.2 to your own experience.

---

### Activity 11.3          *Evidence-based practice and research*

The research findings presented in Table 11.2 are from a longitudinal study conducted between 2000 and 2004. This activity asks you to check whether it is relevant to your current practice.

- Do you think the factors inhibiting confidence are still applicable?
- Do you think the factors developing confidence are still applicable?
- What other factors do you think inhibit confidence in decision-making?
- What other factors do you think develop confidence in decision-making?
- Select two factors inhibiting confidence and identify how to weaken their effect.
- Select two factors developing confidence and identify how to strengthen their effect.

*As these are for your own consideration, no outline answers are given. It might be an idea to discuss the activity with peer group, work colleagues, mentor or supervisor to check out their views on it.*

---

We now focus on developing confidence. In Table 11.2 personal, theoretical and practical factors associated with developing confidence in decision-making seem to combine supportive and challenging elements.

- *Personal factors* – supportive relationships versus 'growing up'.
- *Theoretical factors* – peer support versus picking apart what you say.
- *Practical factors* – trusted team member versus having to deal with situations.

It seems that if we just have the supportive input, we will not learn to 'stand on our own two feet' in making decisions, dealing with situations and explaining, justifying and defending actions. On the other hand, if we just have the challenging input, it will be more difficult to develop confidence in the absence of any perceived support. Balancing contrasting and complementary supportive and challenging experiences appears crucial in developing our confidence in decision-making ability. Hence mentoring needs to balance being supportive and challenging (Standing, 1999). While we are mainly concerned with developing nurses' confidence in clinical decision-making, it can have 'spin-off' effects in our personal lives, too, as the following case study illustrates.

## Case study: Confronting messy housemates

*Mark, a third-year nursing student, was asked how he had developed personally since starting the nursing programme and whether this influenced his decision-making ability. He replied, 'In the past, quite often something will happen and go by and I become aware that I did not act in the way I wanted to because I wasn't confident enough that my intuition was right. I have noticed a change in myself recently. I feel more confident now and it affects my personal life too. For example, some of my housemates are not incredibly diligent with their personal hygiene and I let it go by, but it just got worse. It came to a point where I mentioned it to them. I said they could do what they liked in their rooms but the bathroom and kitchen are for all of us to share so we need to keep them clear of mess for each other's sake. I for one was tired of cleaning up other people's mess before I could get on with what I had to do at the end of a shift. Things did get better afterwards. I don't think I could have done that before I started the programme.'*

The case study illustrates how it takes a certain amount of courage to be self-confident and assertive when we need to be, as others seem to 'step over the line' of acceptable behaviour. Mark's statement is decidedly skewed towards challenging (confronting) as opposed to being supportive, but there is a semblance of support for his housemates' alternative lifestyle in saying 'they can do what they liked in their rooms'. (He was also asking them to be supportive of his efforts to keep shared areas clean and tidy.) Theoretical factors such as a better understanding of personal hygiene, infection control and food poisoning, and practical factors regarding lack of access to or use of basic facilities may have also informed Mark's assessment of the situation. In this sense, confidence in personal decision-making can combine personal, theoretical and practical factors. The next case study refers to nurses' confidence in clinical decision-making.

## Case study: Finding a voice

*Sarah, a third-year nursing student, was asked to reflect on how her understanding of clinical decision-making had developed since commencing the nursing programme. She replied, 'As a first year, you are watching everything in the clinical areas and taking it on-board but you have no voice. In the second year, you get a bit braver and voice opinions about patient care, waiting for support, feedback and confirmation: 'Was I right to say that?' Then, as a third year, you are more knowledgeable; you know that what you are proposing is sound because it is research-based, that we should be going that way in our decision-making, and the voice comes out.'*

In the case study Sarah associated growth in self-confidence with 'finding her voice' in saying what action needs taking and in justifying her decision-making. Sarah alluded to growth in her understanding of clinical practice ('watching everything' and 'taking it on-board') and knowledge of relevant research and how it applied to patient care. In doing so, Sarah integrated personal (brought selves), theoretical (research-based selves), and practical (situationally created selves) factors that develop our confidence in clinical decision-making. In the final case study we revisit Amy (from the first case study in this chapter) and see how her confidence in clinical decision-making has grown.

## Case study: Don't let me die

*Amy has now completed the nursing programme and is waiting for her NMC registration to come through. She no longer lives with mum, as she has got married and set up a new home. She has been working on night duty in a medical unit for the last two months. Benjamin, aged 72, is treated for congestive cardiac failure (weakened heart does not pump efficiently, associated with oedema – build-up of fluid in ankles or, more dangerously, in lungs) and chest infection. Benjamin has medication to regulate heart function, remove excess fluid and fight infection. In spite of this, he is usually very perky when he sees Amy. He likes to impart 'pearls of wisdom', repeatedly telling Amy that the most common phrases in the English language are 'I wish' and 'If only'.*

*One night Benjamin complains he cannot breathe properly. Amy sees he has slipped down the bed and repositions him – with help from an HCA – to elevate and support his back. Amy does this to raise the chest, making breathing easier and reducing the risk of fluid settling in the lungs (pulmonary oedema). Amy checks Benjamin's vital signs and that he has had his medication. Later, he wakes other patients by crying out for help. Amy reports to the clinical manager who instructs her to administer oxygen. Initially it seems to help but then Benjamin complains again. Amy asks the clinical manager if she should call the doctor. The manager tells her they need a good reason to do so and she should try and calm Benjamin down. However, he gets even more distressed and says, 'Don't let me die, Amy'. Amy is sure something is wrong. She examines Benjamin and sees areas of swelling around his chest and neck that crackle and pop when touched. Benjamin says he feels he is being 'strangled' by his own air. Amy decides she needs to call the duty doctor right away, and then informs the clinical manager. The doctor uses a needle to release air trapped under skin (subcutaneous emphysema) that had leaked out of his lungs, and this relieves symptoms. The duty manager tells Amy she made the right call.*

The case study shows how much Amy had grown in confidence since she started the nursing programme. From someone who was dependent on her mum to make everyday decisions for her, she had become autonomous and confident, assessing risks to Benjamin's health, deciding it required urgent medical intervention, and calling the doctor out. In doing so she demonstrated that she had undergone considerable personal and professional development in the space of three years. Her self-confidence increased through what she called 'growing up'. Professional assurance increased as Amy made it her business to keep up to date with nursing research, clinical science, and how this could be applied to patients in her care. Amy combined personal and professional confidence in good interpersonal skills with patients and team members. It was Amy that Benjamin trusted to help him when he was distressed about his breathing problem, and she was instrumental in ensuring the outcome was a positive one. In Table 11.3 Amy's confidence in decision-making is mapped against the conceptions of nursing.

Table 11.3 relates the knowledge, skills and attitudes applied by Amy and the confidence she demonstrated in clinical decision-making to the conceptions of nursing. Activity 11.4 then asks you to use the same format to map out your confidence in clinical decision-making.

| Conceptions of nursing | Confidence in clinical decision-making |
|---|---|
| Caring | Supportive in trying to relieve Benjamin's discomfort |
| Listening and being there | Responsive to Benjamin's calls for help, and attentive |
| Practical procedures | Safely lifting and repositioning to improve breathing, giving oxygen, observing vital signs, assessing breathing problem |
| Knowledge and understanding | Congestive cardiac failure and chest infection nursing care and medical treatment, clinical science, risk assessment |
| Communicating | Establishing good rapport with Benjamin, asking him what was worrying him, advocating medical referral on his behalf |
| Patience | Persevering until solution to problem found, not blaming Benjamin for waking patients, waiting before calling for doctor |
| Teamwork | Working with HCA to reposition Benjamin, reporting change in condition to clinical manager, asking duty doctor to attend |
| Paperwork and electronic record | Recording vital signs, checking medication chart, recording changes in Benjamin's condition and corresponding action |
| Empathising and non-judgemental | Sensing something was wrong: Benjamin was not his usual perky self, he was very distressed and frightened |
| Professional | Prioritising Benjamin's safety, acting autonomously to call duty doctor urgently, and able to justify decision-making |

*Table 11.3: Integrating confidence in clinical decision-making and conceptions of nursing*

## Activity 11.4 — *Decision-making*

Look at how Amy's confidence in clinical decision-making was mapped against the conceptions of nursing in Table 11.3. Identify an incident where you had to find the confidence to deal with a clinical situation. Use the same structure to plot your decision-making and actions. Notice the number and range of knowledge, skills and attitudes you

*continued overleaf . . .*

*continued . . .* •••••••••••••••••••••••••••••••••••••••••••••••••••••••••••••••

have identified. Does this help you to articulate and justify what you do in clinical practice? Does it help you identify areas you would like to develop?

*As this is for your own development no outline answer is given, but it might be useful to discuss your responses with a mentor or supervisor and possibly agree an action plan.*

# Confidence in all types of clinical decision-making

Like accountability (Chapter 10), confidence alone does not tell us how to make decisions, but it enhances every decision we make as we are more effective and patients feel safer if we are confident in what we are doing. Table 11.4 applies confidence to all the decision-making types.

| Decision-making | Examples of applying confidence |
|---|---|
| *Collaborative* | Effective consultation, negotiation and cooperation with patients and team |
| *Observation* | Accurately assess patients' health using all senses, and report concerns |
| *Systematic* | Methodical application of both critical thinking and problem-solving skills |
| *Standardised* | Thorough implementation of NHS Trust procedures and NICE guidelines |
| *Prioritising* | Vigilant, responsive and effective risk assessment and management skills |
| *Experience and intuition* | Intuitively grasp complex situations and how to react to them quickly |
| *Reflective* | Ability to keep clear head, think things through and learn from experience |
| *Ethical sensitivity* | Advocate of patients' rights – informed consent, dignity and confidentiality |
| *Accountability* | Able to explain, justify, defend decision-making with reference to evidence |

*Table 11.4: Confidence in all types of clinical decision-making*

Table 11.4 represents a quick reference guide that summarises what this book is all about. It identifies a wide range of clinical judgement and decision-making types, and associated skills, to help you to be more informed and confident in developing and applying them to patient care. We now take a brief look at how you can continue to develop after becoming a registered nurse.

# How to develop confidence in decision-making as a registered nurse

Throughout your nursing programme you will have had personal tutors and clinical mentors that you can talk to about your personal and professional development. Once you are a registered nurse you have far more responsibilities but fewer opportunities to talk to someone about it. If you do not have any means of ongoing support at work, it can be quite daunting and limits what you learn, as discussing events often helps 'the bell to ring' as you begin to understand more. It is, therefore, highly recommended that you receive clinical supervision that can both support and challenge you in developing your confidence in clinical decision-making further. According to Proctor (1986) clinical supervision has three functions, which complement the personal and professional (theoretical and practical) aspects of confidence discussed earlier.

1. *Supportive* – coping with stress at work (develop personal confidence).
2. *Educational* – developing knowledge and skills (develop theoretical confidence).
3. *Managerial* – monitoring quality of clinical practice (develop practical confidence).

As we have seen in this chapter, all three areas are important in developing confidence in clinical decision-making. Given that nursing practice, healthcare and the nature of health and illness is constantly changing, we need to engage in lifelong learning just to keep up with it. Clinical supervision can make a very useful contribution in this respect, as a way of continuing to develop personal and professional confidence in our judgement and decision-making.

### Chapter summary

This chapter explored the concept of confidence and applied it to clinical decision-making in nursing. A distinction was made between self-confidence and inspiring confidence in others such as patients and team members. It was argued that both are needed since clinical decision-making requires self-assurance or assertiveness but also evidence-based knowledge and practical skills to inspire patients to trust us with their care. Reinharz's three categories of selves (brought, research-based, situationally created) were related to personal, theoretical and practical confidence and highlighted possible personal biases that can be challenged. Factors that inhibit or develop confidence in clinical decision-making were identified with reference to research evidence. Case studies were used to demonstrate a progression in students' confidence over a three-year period and showed how personal, theoretical and practical factors were integrated. Confidence was related to all the other types of decision-making discussed in the book, and a case was made for clinical supervision to help us continue our lifelong learning in professional and personal development after qualifying as a nurse.

## Activities: brief outline answers

### Activity 11.1 Leadership and management (page 179)

You may have included the following points.

*Ensuring safety of all patients*
- Instruct Nathan to return to the unit with the three patients immediately.

*Talking to Nathan about behaviour*
- He exposed his three patients to unnecessary risks and if anything happened, such as one of them having a fit, or wandering off, he would not be able to cope.
- He exposed the remaining patients in the unit to risk because of the reduced staff numbers.
- He should never take patients out without permission.
- He should always report when he is leaving the unit.

## Further reading

**Bach, S and Ellis, P** (2011) *Leadership, Management and Team Working in Nursing.* Exeter: Learning Matters.

Useful information on clinical supervision and the learning environment.

# Glossary

*accountability in clinical decision-making*   being answerable to patients, public, employers, NMC and the law for the consequences of actions, and having to explain, justify or defend your decisions.

*clinical decision-making*   applying clinical judgement to select the best available evidence-based option to control risks and address patients' needs in high quality care you are accountable for.

*clinical judgement*   informed opinion (using intuition, reflection and critical thinking) that relates observation and assessment of patients to identifying and evaluating alternative nursing options.

*collaborative decision-making*   consulting with patients, relatives, nurses, mentors, managers and other health professionals or agencies in order to inform relevant patient-centred decisions.

*confidence in decision-making*   self-assurance from previous experience or achievements and professional assurance (respecting confidentiality, applying evidence-based practice) to inspire patients to trust you to help them, and enable you to explain, justify and defend your decisions.

*critical incidents*   events having a significant impact on you, prompting you to reflect on them.

*critical thinking*   questioning one's own and other's assumptions, addressing gaps in knowledge to achieve aims, challenging illogical or unethical beliefs or practice, evaluating strength of available evidence and presenting a logical, evidence-based argument and defend it when challenged.

*embedded knowledge*   information cues in clinical practice requiring keen observation for detection.

*embodied knowledge*   subconscious accumulation of personal experience drawn on in intuition.

*espoused theories*   concepts, academic knowledge derived from formal learning in university.

*ethical sensitivity in clinical decision-making*   application of ethical principles (do not harm, actions beneficial, respect freedom of choice, fairness to all); for example, patients informed and consent to care, respect confidentiality, break 'bad news' compassionately, and discuss treatment dilemmas.

*evidence*   any kind of information that is used to support reasoning, problem solving, clinical judgement and decision-making, including observations, feedback, policy, theory and research.

*evidence-based practice*   never being satisfied that you 'know it all' and using critical thinking skills to continually search, access, evaluate and apply the most relevant up-to-date sources and types of information to guide clinical judgement/decision-making in giving high quality care.

*experience and intuition in decision-making*   recognising similarities and differences between current and previous situations and being guided by what seemed effective before (and learning from any earlier mistakes) or realising you lack the necessary experience to make a decision.

*hermeneutic phenomenology*   involves the researcher seeking to elicit person's perceptions of interacting with others and how they make sense of their lived experience, without imposing his/her own agenda.

*information processing*   ability to take in sensory, verbal, non-verbal and numerical data, then interpret and classify, store in short- or long-term memory, and retrieve and apply it as needed.

*nursing*   promoting health, prevention or recovery from illness or injury, adaptation to disability, or dignity in facing death in patient-centred care applying bio–psycho–social–spiritual knowledge, skills and ethical values to safe, effective judgement, decisions and evidence-based practice.

*nursing theory*   philosophy or model defining interrelationships between concepts of 'humans/environment/health/nursing' to explain values, vital knowledge or skills, and nurses' role.

*observation in clinical decision-making*   continuous use of senses (sight, hearing, touch or smell) to assess patients' bio–psycho–social–spiritual well-being, check if they need assistance, monitor vital signs, review results of investigations, record response to treatment, and report concerns.

*patient/person-centred care*   tailoring care that is relevant and responsive to patient's needs by identifying their preferences, explaining options, and enabling them to make informed decisions.

*prioritising in decision-making*   risk assessment and management to target care on those with life-threatening illness or injury before others, a patient's urgent needs before non-urgent ones, health promotion for vulnerable groups, and avoiding causing harm to patients in healthcare settings.

*problem solving*   dissatisfaction with current situation prompts the use of critical thinking skills to systematically assess and identify problem, plan, implement action, and evaluate outcome.

*reflective decision-making*   reviewing events as they occur (reflection-in-action) to identify and choose best option or to review past (reflection-on-action) for insights to inform future practice.

*reflexivity*   critical self-examination of the logic and evidence for what we think is true by being open about our potential biases, assuming our interpretations may be wrong and testing them.

*standardised clinical decision-making*   application of NHS Trust policies, procedures and agreed care plans plus evidence-based (NICE) clinical guidelines and assessment tools to guide nursing interventions.

*systematic clinical decision-making*   using critical thinking and problem-solving skills to identify/assess problems, set goals/make plans, deliver nursing care and evaluate outcome, revising as needed.

*theories-in-use*   assumptions, custom and practice derived from informal work-based learning.

*theory–practice gap*   mismatch between what nurses are taught and what they actually do.

# References

Alfaro-LeFevre, R (2009) *Nursing Process: A tool for critical thinking* (7th edn). Philadelphia, PA: Lippincott Williams & Wilkins.

Argyris, C and Schön, D (1974) *Theory in Practice: Increasing personal effectiveness*. Massachusetts: Addison Wesley.

Ahluwalia, RS, Johal, N, Kourief, C et al. (2006) The surgical risk of suprapubic catheter insertion and long term sequelae. *Annals Royal College of Surgeons*, 88(2): 210–13.

Bach, A and Grant, S (2009) *Communication and Interpersonal Skills for Nurses*. Exeter: Learning Matters.

BBC (2010) Tetraplegic man's life support turned off by mistake. Online at www.bbc.co.uk/news/uk-england-wiltshire-11595485

Beauchamp, T and Childress, J (1989) *Principles of Biomedical Ethics*. Oxford: Oxford University Press.

Benner, P (1984) *From Novice to Expert*. Menlo Park, CA: Addison-Wesley.

Bloom, B (1956) *Taxonomy of Educational Objectives – Book 1 The cognitive domain*. London: Longman.

Campbell, H, Hotchkiss, R, Bradshaw, N. and Porteous, M. (1998) Integrated care pathways. *BMJ (British Medical Journal)*, 316 (7125): 133–7.

Cancer Research UK (2009) Breast cancer statistics: key facts. Available online at http://info.cancer researchuk.org/cancerstats/types/breast.

Cancer Research UK (2010) Prostate cancer statistics: key facts. Available online at http://info.cancer researchuk.org/cancerstats/types/prostate.

Chambers (2010) *Chambers 21st Century Dictionary*. Available online at www.chambersharrap.co.uk.

Clark, J (2006) 30th anniversary commentary on Henderson, V (1978) The concept of nursing. *Journal of Advanced Nursing*, 3, 113–30.

Corcoran-Perry, S and Narayan, S (1995) Clinical decision-making, in Snyder, M and Mirr, MP (eds) *Advanced Nursing Practice*. New York: Springer.

DH (Department of Health) (2000) *The NHS Plan*. London: HMSO.

DH (2006a) *Expert Patients Programme*. London: HMSO.

DH (2006b) *Our Health, Our Care, Our Say: A new direction for community services*. London: HMSO.

DH (2008) *High Quality Care for All: NHS Next Step Review final report*. London: HMSO.

DH (2009) *The NHS Constitution*. London: HMSO.

DH (2010a) *National Child Measurement Programme*. London: HMSO.

DH (2010b) *NHS Outcomes Framework*. London: HMSO.

DH (2010c) *Equity and Excellence: Liberating the NHS*. London: HMSO.

Ellis, P. (2010) *Evidence-based Practice in Nursing*. Exeter: Learning Matters.

Evidence Based Nursing Practice (2003) The hierarchy of evidence. Online at www.ebnp.co.uk/The%20 Hierarchy%20of%20Evidence.htm.

Fawcett, J (2005) *Contemporary Nursing Knowledge*. Philadelphia, PA: FA Davies.

Fleming, K and Fenton, M (2002) Making sense of research evidence to inform decision-making, in Thompson, C and Dowding, D (eds) *Clinical Decision Making and Judgement in Nursing*. Edinburgh: Churchill Livingstone.

Gardner, H (1983) *Frames of Mind: The theory of multiple intelligences*. New York: Basic Books.

Gawande, A (2010) *The Checklist Manifesto: How to get things right*. London: Profile Books.

Gonzalez, J and Wagenaar, R (2003) *Tuning Educational Structures in Europe: Final report pilot project – Phase 1*. Bilbao: University of Deusto.

Griffith, JW and Christensen, PJ (1982) *Nursing Process: Application of theories, frameworks and models*. St Louis, MO: Mosby.

Griffith, R and Tengnah, C (2010) *Law and Professional Issues in Nursing*. Exeter: Learning Matters.

Hammond, KR (1996) *Human Judgement and Social Policy: Irreducible uncertainty, inevitable error, unavoidable injustice*. New York: Oxford University Press.

Haynes, AB, Weisner, TG, Berry, WR et al. (2009) A surgical safety checklist to reduce morbidity and mortality in a global population. *New England Journal of Medicine*, 360: 491–9.

Hek, G and Moule, P (2006) *Making Sense of Research* (3rd edn). London: Sage.

Henderson, V (1966) *The Nature of Nursing*. New York: Macmillan.

Hernanz-Schulman, M (2003) Infantile hypertrophic pyloric stenosis. *Radiology*, 227: 319–31.

Heron, J (1989) *Six Category Intervention Analysis*. Guildford: Human Potential Resource Group, University of Surrey.

Higgs, J and Titchen, A (2001) *Practice Knowledge and Expertise*. Oxford: Butterworth Heinemann.

Howatson-Jones, L (2010) *Reflective Practice in Nursing*. Exeter: Learning Matters.

ICN (International Council of Nurses) (2009) *ICN Framework of Competencies for the Nurse Specialist*. Geneva: ICN.

Jasper, M (2006) *Professional Development, Reflection and Decision making*. Oxford: Blackwell.

Kipling, R (1902) I keep six honest serving men, in Kipling, R. *The Elephant's Child* (Just so stories). Available online at www.kipling.org.uk/poems_serving.htm.

Kolb, DA (1984) *Experiential Learning*. Englewood Cliffs, NJ: Prentice-Hall.

Koopmans, M (1997) Schizophrenia and the family: double bind theory revisited. Available online at www.goertzel.org/dynapsyc/1997/Koopmans.html.

Leininger, M (1985) Transcultural nursing care: diversity and universality. *Nursing and Health Care*, 6: 209–12.

Middleton, S, Barnett, J and Reeves, D (2001) What is an integrated care pathway? *Evidence Based Medicine* 3(3): 1–7. Available at www.medicine.ox.ac.uk/bandolier/painres/dowload/whatis/What_is_ICP.pdf

NHS (National Health Service) (2010) What's your BMI? Available online at www.nhs.uk/LiveWell/loseweight/Pages/BodyMassIndex.aspx.

NHS Information Centre (2009) Statistics on alcohol, England 2009. Available online at www.ic.nhs.uk/pubs/alcohol09.

NICE (National Institute for Health and Clinical Excellence) (2005) *Violence: The short term management of disturbed/violent behaviour in inpatient psychiatric settings and emergency departments*. London: NICE.

NICE (2007a) *How to Change Practice: Understand, identify and overcome barriers to change.* London: NICE.

NICE (2007b) *Acutely Ill Patients in Hospital: Recognition and response to acute illness in hospital.* London: NICE.

NICE (2009) *Depression: The treatment and management of depression in adults.* National Clinical Practice Guideline 90. Available online at www.nice.org.uk/nicemedia/live/12329/45896/45896.pdf.

NICE (2010a) *Alcohol Use Disorders: Preventing harmful drinking.* Public Health Guidance 24. London: NICE.

NICE (2010b) *Chest Pain of Recent Onset.* Clinical Guideline 95. London: NICE.

NICE (2011) *Generalised Anxiety Disorder and Panic Disorder (With or Without Agoraphobia) in Adults.* National Clinical Guideline No. 113. London: NICE.

Nightingale, F (1860) *Notes on Nursing: What it is and what it is not.* New York: Appleton.

NMC (Nursing and Midwifery Council) (2008) *The Code: Standards of conduct, performance and ethics for nurses and midwives.* London: NMC.

NMC (2009a) *Guidance on Professional Conduct for Nursing and Midwifery Students.* London: NMC.

NMC (2009b) *Record Keeping: Guidance for nurses and midwives.* London: NMC.

NMC (2010a) *Standards for Pre-registration Nursing Education.* London: NMC.

NMC (2010b) www.nmc-uk.org/Hearings/Hearings-and-outcomes

NPSA (National Patient Safety Agency) (2007) *Safer Care for the Acutely Ill Patient: Learning from incidents.* 5th Report from the Patient Safety Observatory. Available online at www.npsa.nhs.uk.

Office for National Statistics (2006) *Mortality Statistics – Series DH2 no. 3.* London: HMSO.

Olver, K (2007) Ten critical de-escalation skills. Online at www.thefreelibrary.com/Ten%20Critical%20De-Escalation%20Skills-a01073764673.

Orem, D (1980) *Nursing: Concepts of Practice.* New York: McGraw-Hill.

Parse, RR (1992) Human becoming: Parse's theory of nursing. *Nursing Science Quarterly*, 5(1): 35–42.

Peplau, H (1952) *Interpersonal Relations in Nursing.* New York: Putman and Sons.

Powell, H and Murray, G (2004) Staff perceptions of community learning disability nurses' role. *Nursing Times*, 100(19): 40.

Proctor, B (1986) Supervision: a cooperative exercise in accountability, in Marken, M. and Payne, M. (eds) *Enabling and Ensuring: Supervision in Practice.* Leicester: National Youth Bureau, Council for Education and Training in Youth and Community Work.

Pronovost, P, Needham, D, Berenholtz, S et al. (2006) An intervention to reduce catheter-related bloodstream infections in the ICU. *New England Journal of Medicine*, 355: 2725–32.

RCN (Royal College of Nursing) (2003) *Defining Nursing.* London: RCN.

RCN (2010) Principles of nursing practice. Online at www.rcn.org.uk/development/practice/principles.

Reinharz, S (1997) Who am I? The need for a variety of selves in the field, in Hertz, R. (ed.) *Reflexivity and Voice.* Thousand Oaks, CA: Sage.

Rogers, EM (1962) *Diffusion of Innovations.* Glencoe: Free Press.

Roper, N, Logan, WW and Tierney, AJ (2000) *The Roper-Logan-Tierney Model of Nursing: Based on Activities of Living.* Edinburgh: Churchill Livingstone.

Roy, C (1980) *Introduction to Nursing: An adaptation model.* Englewood Cliffs, NJ: Prentice-Hall.

Rycroft-Malone, J, Seers, K, Titchen, A et al. (2004) What counts as evidence-based practice? *Journal of Advanced Nursing*, 47: 81–90.

Saunders, JB, Aasland, O.G., Babor, T.F. et al. (1993) Development of the Alcohol Use Disorders Identification Test (AUDIT): WHO collaborative project on early detection of persons with harmful alcohol consumption. *Addiction*, 88: 349–62.

Schön, DA (1983) *The Reflective Practitioner.* New York: Basic Books.

Snyder, M (1995) Advance practice within a nursing paradigm, in Snyder, M and Mirr, MP (eds) *Advanced Nursing Practice.* New York: Springer.

Standing, M (1999) Developing a Supportive/Challenging and Reflective/Competency Education (SCARCE) mentoring model and discussing its relevance to nurse education. *Mentoring and Tutoring*, 6(3): 3–17.

Standing, M (2005) Perceptions of clinical decision-making on a developmental journey from student to staff nurse. Unpublished PhD Thesis. Canterbury: University of Kent.

Standing, M (2007) Clinical decision-making skills on the developmental journey from student to registered nurse: a longitudinal inquiry. *Journal of Advanced Nursing*, 60(3): 257–69.

Standing, M (2010) Perceptions of clinical decision-making: a matrix model, in Standing, M (ed.) *Clinical Judgement and Decision Making: Nursing and interprofessional healthcare.* Maidenhead: Open University Press.

Standing, M and Standing, MRJ (2010) Reflexive-pragmatism: logic, practicality, rigour and relevance, in Standing, M (ed.) *Clinical Judgement and Decision Making: Nursing and interprofessional healthcare.* Maidenhead: Open University Press.

St John Ambulance, St Andrews Ambulance Association and British Red Cross Society (2009) *First Aid Manual* (9th edn). London: Dorling Kindersley.

Trower, P, Casey, A and Dryden, W (1988) *Cognitive-behavioural Counselling in Action.* London: Sage.

Wallace, P (2001) Patients with alcohol problems: simple questioning is the key to effective identification and management. *British Journal of General Practice*, 51: 172–3.

Watson, J (1988) *Nursing: Human science and human care.* New York: National League for Nursing.

WHO (World Health Organization) (1948) *Official Records of the World Health Organization.* Geneva: WHO.

WHO (2009) *Surgical Safety Checklist.* Geneva: WHO.

Yura, H and Walsh, MB (1973) *The Nursing Process.* New York: Appleton-Century-Crofts.

# Index